Making partnerships work in community care

A guide for practitioners in housing, health and social services

Robin Means, Maria Brenton, Lyn Harrison and Frances Heywood

First published in Great Britain in 1997 by

The Policy Press
University of Bristol
Rodney Lodge
Grange Road
Bristol BS8 4EA

Telephone: (+44) (0)117 973 8797
Fax: (+44) (0)117 973 7308
E-mail: tpp@bris.ac.uk
Website: http://www.bris.ac.uk/Publications/TPP

In association with the Department of Health and the Department of the Environment, Transport and the Regions.

© Crown copyright

ISBN 1 86134 058 3

Robin Means is Reader in Social Gerontology, Maria Brenton is a Visiting Research Fellow, Lyn Harrison is a Senior Lecturer and Frances Heywood is a Research Fellow, all based at the School for Policy Studies, University of Bristol.

The Policy Press works to counter discrimination on grounds of gender, race, disability, age and sexuality.

Cover and text designed by Qube Design Associates, Bristol.
Printed in Great Britain by H. Charlesworth & Co Ltd, Huddersfield.

Acknowledgements

This workbook has been made possible through the help and advice received from numerous sources. The first of these were our service user consultants namely Viv Lindow, John Winfield and the group of older service users from the Wiltshire and Swindon Users' Network who all combined a commitment to principles and values with a practical emphasis upon the need to improve joint working on the ground. Further advice was received from the Practitioner Panel who spent two separate days with us as well as sending in numerous good practice suggestions. In addition we would like to thank Louise Russell (Age Concern, England) for her input into Module Two and Pat Turton (University of Bristol) for help with Module Five. Equally important was the supportive advice from the Steering Group, and in particular from the two lead officers for the workbook, namely Amanda Edwards (Department of Health) and Peter Faherty (Department of the Environment, Transport and the Regions). In addition numerous individuals took the time to comment upon earlier drafts and in this respect we would particularly like to thank Mark Brangwyn and Geoff Matthews from the local authority associations. We would like to acknowledge the copyright permission to use various extracts received from the Age Concern (England), the Audit Commission, the Chartered Institute of Housing, the King's Fund Institute, the Mental Health Foundation and the Joseph Rowntree Foundation. Finally we would like to thank Linda Price for her secretarial support to this project and staff at The Policy Press for their speedy and efficient help in the production of the workbook.

Members of the Steering Group

Reba Bhaduri (Department of Health)
Amanda Edwards (Department of Health)
Peter Faherty (Department of the Environment, Transport and the Regions)
Derek Goring (Department of Health)
Chris Gostick (NHS Executive)
Judith Harrison (The Housing Corporation)
Andy Ludlow/Catherine McAdam (Haringey Social Services)
Oliver McGeachy (National Users and Carers Group)
Jo McTavish (Hyde Housing Association)
Bridget Ogden (Department of Health)
Julian Oliver (Department of Health)

Practitioner Panel

Carol Barrett-Williams (London Borough of Haringey)
Jackie Bates (Terrance Higgins Trust)
Melody Carter (Southmead Hospital, Bristol)
Steve Cody (London Borough of Lambeth)
Jane Cook (Camden and Islington Health Authority)
Sue Forber (Wiltshire County Council)
Kate Frost (York Housing Association)
Abi Gilbert (Community Practitioners and Health Visitors Association)
Meg Groves (City of Bradford Metropolitan Council)
Simon Hood (Salford Borough Council)
Helen Keats (Portsmouth City Council)
Donna Kelly (Riverside Housing Association)
Susanna McCorry (Friendship Group)
Mary McGowan (London Borough of Camden)
John Molloy (Salford Borough Council)
Nick Murphy (Housing Advice Centre, Eastbourne)
Ann Palmer (London and Quadrant Housing Trust)
Teresa Parker (Housing 21)
Christine Peacock (City of Bradford Metropolitan Council)
Lawrence Santcross (Stonham Housing Association)
Ian Sissling (St Anne's Shelter and Housing Action, Leeds)
Mary Tam (London Borough of Haringey)
Jenny Treadwell (United Bristol Health Trust)
Lesley Wheal (Tonbridge and Malling Home Improvment Agency)

Contents

introduction

Aims of the workbook

Community care means providing the services and support which people ... need to be able to live as independently as possible in their own home, or in 'homely' settings in the community. (Department of Health [1989] *Caring for people: community care in the next decade and beyond*, London: HMSO, p 3)

Central and local government are committed to the value of social care and recognise that the housing dimension can be crucial in the success of health and community care policy and practice. The local social services and housing authorities have statutory responsibility for the assessment and delivery of services for people who require community care services. Central government has recently produced *Housing and community care: establishing a strategic framework* (Department of Health/Department of the Environment, 1997) in order to promote joint working.

This workbook, designed to assist care managers and practitioners, is intended to enable joint working between agencies to develop and flourish at the operational level and will assist those responsible for supporting individuals in the statutory and independent sectors to better appreciate the respective roles of housing, health and social care agencies. Such individuals will also need to know the current policy and practice of their local authorities as set out in community care plans and housing strategy statements which are prepared and published annually. The Housing Corporation regional office, local Health Authorities and, increasingly local general practitioners (GPs), also prepare purchasing plans for the locality. These statements and objectives provide the context and objectives for community care and will indicate the opportunities for services in each locality. The absence of appropriate support should also be identified as a basis for informing future plans and purchasing decisions and may also assist in the development of joint commissioning between agencies.

The key to success in the provision of community care can often be the strength of local partnerships for action and the commitment of staff to making appropriate arrangements for the support of individuals.

The overall aims of the workbook are as follows:

- to encourage and facilitate a partnership approach to joint working at the operational level, across housing, health and social services;

- to encourage practitioners to carry out their work in a way which includes service users and carers as partners;

- to demonstrate why joint working is essential even if it is difficult to achieve in practice;

- to provide specific guidance and innovative practice examples in such areas as care management, homelessness, home improvement and adaptation and hospital discharge.

Importance of home and housing

It's a lot better to live on your own. It's important that people with learning disabilities have the right to their own home and their own key and live by themselves. (Mental Health Foundation [1996] *Building expectations*, London: Mental Health Foundation)

Mr Jones: "It's a place of retreat really".
Mrs Jones: " ... and home's always been a place where you want to go back to, however humble it is. Even when we go to town, we're still glad, well I am, to get back.... It's a place of our own. (Langan et al [1996] *Maintaining independence in later life: older people speaking*, Oxford: Anchor, p 6)

"Having a beautifully adapted home has given Liz and I the platform to live out our visions together." (John Winfield, consultant adviser to the authors of the workbook)

Who is the workbook for?

The workbook is primarily aimed at first-line managers (team leaders, etc) in social services, housing and health agencies. This includes not just statutory agencies but also many private and voluntary sector organisations including those working for organisations controlled by service users and/or disabled people. The workbook will also be invaluable to individual field-level and front-line staff involved in providing assessments and assisting in the provision of services for people with learning disabilities and mental health problems, elderly people with support needs, physically disabled people, people with AIDS and HIV infection, and people with alcohol and drugs problems. All need a broad knowledge of how local agencies can work together.

The workbook does *not* address issues of joint working between housing, health and social services relating to young people and the 1989 Childrens Act. However, many of the principles discussed and outlined are relevant to all aspects of joint working at the operational level between these agencies.

Outline of the workbook

Module One of the workbook looks at the general challenge posed by joint working. It stresses the need for joint working to be underpinned by clear principles which stress that joint working is about delivering user-driven services. **Module One** outlines both the obstacles to effective collaboration but also how these might be overcome. Since joint working is often undermined by a lack of understanding between agencies, the Module concludes by providing a snapshot of the policy context within which housing, health and social services operate. **Module Two** develops this further by focusing upon the need for operational staff to map each others' organisations and to develop a resource file. Key mapping questions are outlined

for each of social services, health and housing.

Module Three shifts the focus to assessment and care management. It looks at the questions which housing staff need to ask about care management and which questions social services staff need to ask about housing. It then goes on to look at the specific issues raised by homeless people and by vulnerable tenants. The second half of the Module looks at the monitoring and review of care and support arrangements as well as the development of detailed joint procedures and protocols. Joint assessments, monitoring and review are seen as extremely positive developments but ones requiring clarity on when and how to exchange information about individuals.

Module Four looks at home adaptation and home improvement. Warm, safe, comfortable and well adapted housing can make a major contribution to community care and this Module argues that tackling poor and disabling housing requires cooperation between housing, social services and health. It looks at the action which can be taken by each of these agencies and how this relates to the housing renewal grants system and other sources of help. Examples of cooperation are given in terms of (i) making information available; (ii) assessment and specification; (iii) delivering a swift and user friendly service; and (iv) ensuring that building work is backed up by support services.

Module Five and **Module Six** focus centrally upon the role of health professionals. **Module Five** looks at housing agencies and primary healthcare teams in terms of their need to work jointly (i) during the process of housing allocation; (ii) in enabling individuals to 'stay put'; and (iii) during the care management assessment of individuals who have health and housing needs. The Module outlines what primary healthcare staff need to understand about housing and what housing staff need to know about GPs and primary healthcare teams. The second half of the Module considers common problems and potential solutions, and it concludes by offering a series of innovative practice examples.

Module Six looks at hospital admission and discharge. It begins by outlining the policy context, including the approach advocated by the hospital discharge workbook. It goes on to consider what hospital ward and social services staff need to know about housing, and what housing staff need to know about hospitals and hospital discharge. General issues and potential solutions faced by all the key agencies are outlined. The second half of the Module deals with the hospital discharge of people with mental health problems. The specific housing issues and questions raised are addressed and innovative practice examples profiled.

Using the workbook

The workbook is not designed to be read from cover to cover. We would, however, encourage all users of the workbook to look at **Module One** even though some will feel they are already well aware of the challenges of joint working. **Module Two** on mapping is designed not to be necessarily followed page by page, but to stimulate operational staff and their managers to clarify what they need to know about partner agencies and to ensure that this is collected in an accessible form.

The remaining Modules are designed to be used and drawn upon as and when appropriate. The Contents page is presented in a very detailed format in order to facilitate the location of appropriate sections. Some overlap has been built into the Modules in order to reduce the amount of cross-referencing required between them.

The challenge of joint working

module one

Objectives

1 To show that joint working is essential to the provision of responsive services to the people who use them.

2 To define the different dimensions of joint working and explain why joint working can be difficult to achieve.

3 To provide guidance on how joint working can be supported and progressed.

4 To develop the capacity of staff in housing, health and social services to understand each others' organisations.

Why work together?

- **It solves problems and offers a better service:** individuals have needs which span community care, health and housing, and hence an effective response to their needs requires a commitment to collaboration from a wide range of professionals.

- **It saves time and money:** a failure to collaborate not only reduces the quality and appropriateness of services received by service users but also imposes costs upon professionals. Expensive residential care may need to be offered because of a failure to support people in their own homes. Misunderstandings and lack of cooperation between professionals can result in care package breakdown, numerous case conferences, etc. Joint working eliminates gaps and overlaps in service provision.

- **Joint working is happening:** health, housing and social services professionals are constantly in touch with each other and the importance of working together is stressed increasingly by central government. Since joint working needs to happen, it makes sense for professionals to improve their joint working skills.

Establishing key principles

Joint working is not an end in itself but a means to help facilitate the provision of appropriate services. There is considerable agreement about the principles which service users wish to see underpin the development and operational delivery of housing, health and social care services.

- **Full membership of society:** people with housing, care and support needs wish to be full members of the communities, towns and villages in which they live. The achievement of independence and choice requires tackling the barriers they face in society – people may have impairments but what actually disables them are lack of opportunities to engage as full citizens of society. This underlines that professionals need to consider the overall quality of life of service users, and how this relates to their need for housing and support.

- **Equal opportunities:** it is crucial that all people requiring services are assessed in ways which do not restrict access to appropriate housing and support services, and hence services need to reflect the diversity of local communities. Professionals need to be willing to tackle discrimination on the grounds of age, gender, race, disability and sexuality.

- **Access to mainstream housing and mainstream services:** the preference of most people is for access to mainstream housing and mainstream services which must develop the flexibility to respond to individual requirements.

- **Combining appropriate housing with appropriate support:** inadequate housing can undermine a good support package while a poor support package can lead to a failure to establish independent living, despite the availability of adequate housing. A common problem is that failure to supply appropriate support to someone who has moved into 'ordinary' housing can lead to a drift back to more institutional type provision which may well offer a level of support not required by the individual.

- **An appropriate housing solution?:** the appropriateness of accommodation for someone may depend on where it is in relation to shops, buses, work, meaningful activities and support networks. These can be as important as the physical characteristics of the house or flat itself. The importance to housing applicants of such issues as personal safety and noise needs to be recognised as legitimate.

- **'People don't fit the categories':** many traditional combinations of housing and support tend to produce schemes targeted at discrete categories of impairment (mental health, learning disability, frail elders, etc) or social situation (women 'at risk' of domestic violence, ex-offenders, etc). The challenge faced by operational staff is how to offer creative user-driven responses to individual needs and preferences rather than to 'slot' people into available provision.

- **Partnership with users and carers:** increasingly, service users and carers want a partnership with professionals both through collective input to service development and at the level of individual housing and personal assistance arrangements. Professionals should be willing to work with advocates where necessary in order to achieve this. At the operational level, one outcome of partnership may be a changed role for the professional through the introduction of direct payment schemes by which individuals can 'buy in' their own personal assistance requirements.

- **Sharing of client information and confidentiality:** service users and carers wish to see a wide spectrum of professionals working together to help them obtain the right combination of

services. This requires a willingness to share information. It is thus crucial that a working together strategy for housing and community care includes a clear policy on information sharing between agencies and the staff working for them, and this policy needs to include a consideration of issues of confidentiality and privacy.

The challenge of joint working

The above principles underline that service users and carers want a coherent and coordinated response to their housing and support needs which is driven by their needs and preferences. As a result, operational staff in housing, health and social services need to maximise their skills at joint working. Part of the challenge is that joint working covers a wide range of activities:

- **Understanding each other:** good joint working is not always about literally working together! It is about different professionals understanding each other's agencies and so being able to advise individuals about how these agencies might be able to help them. It is about having sufficient knowledge to know when a joint assessment is required because of the complexity of the housing and support issues to be tackled. An understanding of the legislation and financial frameworks of each agency is also helpful.

- **Cooperation:** this reflects a willingness of professionals to assist each other on a day-to-day basis in a constructive and positive manner.

- **Collaboration:** this is when professionals work together with another or others on a joint project, joint initiative or shared case.

- **Coordination:** this involves an attempt to integrate different professionals into the achievement of some agreed objectives. This will often take a written form through the development of **joint protocols** to guide operational staff.

- **Networks:** informal groupings of professionals who meet together to exchange views and to develop cooperation are increasingly common.

- **Partnership:** this is often taken to refer to a much more formal arrangement than a network in which there is clear commitment from one or more organisations to work together on a joint initiative, although it can also be used, as in this workbook, as a more general reference to joint working.

Overcoming obstacles

The obstacles to joint working appear to be the following:

- **Loss of autonomy:** joint working requires organisations and individuals to give up some autonomy to act independently, and they may lose some ability to set and control their own agenda and priorities.

- **The costs of joint working:** good joint working requires that each agency and professional spend time and energy on developing and maintaining relationships with staff from other organisations. It should be remembered that service users also face these costs when involved in joint working as full partners with professionals.

- **Stereotypes:** housing, health and social services professionals often hold negative stereotypes about each other. People requiring services and professionals also hold stereotypes about each other. The more entrenched the stereotypes, the harder it will be to develop joint working.

Professional stereotypes

Housing on social services

There is a stereotyped image of the social worker as young and freshly qualified, straight from school via college, without any practical experience, who would be entirely subjective and idealistic about clients and will seek all manner of handouts and special treatment for them without ever expecting them to stand on their own two feet. (Evidence from an Institute of Housing Sub-Committee submitted to the 1982 Barclay Committee)

Social services on housing

"I am not saying that they are a lot of heartless villains. I just think they are conditioned and they have little scope to do anything other than reach their targets in terms of rent arrears." (Social worker, quoted in Clapham and Franklin, [1994] *The Housing Management contribution to community care*, CHRUS Research Report, University of Glasgow)

- **Cultural differences:** health, housing and social services may hold stereotypes about each other but equally there are real and very important cultural differences in terms of how they understand and respond to need. These cultural differences include the use of jargon particular to each profession.

- **Agreement about roles and responsibilities:** if organisations and professionals disagree over their respective roles, responsibilities and competencies, then this is likely to be an obstacle to effective joint working at the local level.

- **Misunderstandings:** professionals often have only limited knowledge about other professional groups or other organisations with which they wish to liaise and work with. They simply misunderstand the priorities, organisational structures, cultures and working practices of potential collaborative partners, and how this relates to very real statutory differences between housing, health and social services.

Moving forward

However, there is growing understanding about how to foster and support joint working despite the obstacles just outlined. Key elements are:

• **Backing from senior managers:** joint working at the operational level between health, housing and social services must be supported by senior managers at all levels in order to maximise its legitimacy, and to ensure support and encouragement when difficulties are encountered. At the same time, many of the best initiatives originate from field-level staff.

• **Identify objectives and gain for *all* participants:** it is crucial to be clear about what you are attempting to achieve in any joint working initiative. What are your priorities and how does this relate to the resources at your disposal? It is equally important to recognise that all collaborative partners need tangible gains for their own organisation. Joint working initiatives which only meet the objectives of the instigator are likely to fail. Thus, service users are likely to remain committed to joint working with professionals only if they see this as contributing to better services.

• **Mapping:** because joint working can be undermined by misunderstanding, mutual ignorance and stereotypes, mapping is a pivotal activity in terms of identifying the structures, the priorities and the key actors of the organisations you hope to work with. Such information can provide the 'raw data' to develop an implementation strategy for achieving your objectives (see **Module Two**).

A checklist for developing networks

1 Clarify objectives
• Be clear as to what your aims and objectives are.
• Identify priorities and ordering of those priorities.
• Have a clear idea as to what resources are available to you in terms of time, money and skills and identify areas where it will be necessary or desirable to fill gaps or adjust plans.
• Try and be clear as to what strategies are available to you, eg, can you tempt people to participate with a budget, do you have the authority to insist?

2 Mapping the environment
• Identify and map out the relevant agencies and organisations.
• Get a feel for the priorities of these key agencies.
• Identify key policy makers and resource holders, and their attitude to your policy area.
• Identify fellow enthusiasts and whether or not they share your approach or philosophy towards the policy area.
• Identify potential collaborators, ie, the right people in the right positions in the right organisations.

3 Implementation
• Identify the appropriate tactics to achieve your strategy in the light of the objectives and the environment.
• Try and anticipate the likely areas of tension and problems that might obstruct or frustrate your intentions.
• Identify the resources or opportunities available that might promote your project, ie, identifying and meeting a training need.
• Try to build in some possibility of evaluation so that you can see whether you are heading towards your goal, and some mechanism for feeding back the results of any evaluation into your work plan.

- **Identify participants:** by combining clarity about objectives with maps of local actors it is possible to identify who needs to participate in any piece of joint working and why.

- **Build up trust:** part of any implementation strategy needs to include a judgement about the level and types of joint working to aim for. The general message is that collaborative partners should work in the first instance on modest tasks with modest objectives where there has been a past history of conflict and distrust. Success from such ventures creates the platform to go for more challenging initiatives in the future.

- **Incentives:** one mechanism for encouraging joint working is the use of incentives. The offer of 'free' places on joint training courses, the 'free' use of meeting rooms and the recognition of networking activity in workloads are just some examples of possible ways of enticing and supporting collaborative initiatives.

- **Develop a collaborative culture:** as well as key individuals such as senior managers, team leaders or committed field-level staff persuading others of the need for joint working, there is a need to develop a collaborative culture to be shared by a wide range of staff across agencies and based on a commitment to working in partnership with service users and carers. *(See table opposite.)*

Don't be afraid to learn

Professional training rarely covers other sections adequately, and placements all too often fail to provide relevant experience of all the key agencies. The whole area of health, housing and community care is genuinely complicated and so a complete understanding of all three sectors is impossible. The important point is that if you are a professional with a detailed knowledge of your specialist area you should not be deterred from collaborative working by feelings of incompetence and inadequacy. You need to be encouraged to learn, and should not be afraid to make occasional mistakes.

Understanding housing, social services and health

The previous sections of this Module have stressed how joint working is often undermined by a lack of mutual understanding and this highlights the need for an appreciation of the context within which housing, social services and health agencies are operating. A 'snapshot' of core trends and developments follows.

Joint training

Hampshire Social Services Department and Portsmouth Housing Department have run a joint training programme for operational staff with the following objectives:

- to understand each other's role and responsibility;

- to promote good practice;

- to improve (quality) of service;

- to assist the development of joint/complementary processes.

The most effective component of the training was found to be staff discussing their different roles and responsibilities in small groups.

Towards a collaborative culture

The user involvement spectrum	Information for service users and carers	Group consultation with service users and carers
Providing information: how and where decisions are taken and by whom? what services are available and how else could needs be met?	Must be widely available (eg, post offices, libraries, GP surgeries)	Offer training to service users and carers
Individual consultation: individual service users expressing their own needs and how they think these should be met	Easy to read and understand, and hence tested out by reader panels of service users and carers	Use service users and carers to train staff on how to involve non-professionals in meetings
Group consultation: groups of existing or potential service users can be consulted about what kind of services are needed	Available in a wide range of languages	Hold meetings in accessible venues
Joint working: service users working in partnership with professionals on, for instance, writing service specifications or setting quality assurance measures	Translation facilities must be available where no translated form available	Avoid jargon
Delegated control: where statutory agencies delegate control over key decisions or services themselves to individuals or to user-led organisations	Available in non-written form (Braille, tape, etc)	Give adequate time for feedback from service users and carers on proposals
	Clear information needs to be backed up by easy to use forms	Ensure service users and carers are fully informed of action taken after consultation

Source: The first column draws upon work from d'Aboville (1994) *Promoting user involvement*, London: King's Fund. Reproduced by kind permission from the King's Fund.

Housing

1 Many people want to own their own homes and owner-occupation is now the dominant tenure. Alongside this the government is committed to supporting efficiently run social and private rented sectors.

2 The work of housing authorities (metropolitan authorities, district councils and London boroughs) has broadened and diversified in recent years:

i) they have developed their enabling and strategic role;
ii) some local authorities have delegated their housing management services to an external organisation such as a private sector contractor, a managing agent or a tenant management organisation;
iii) some local authorities have transferred some or all of their housing stock usually to registered social landlords which include housing associations (transfer has often been in the form of large-scale voluntary transfer or LSVT; by early 1997, there were over 50 LSVTs managing around 250,000 socially rented homes).

3 Social housing now:

i) houses a high proportion of 'vulnerable' households;
ii) is allocated more on the basis of need.

4 The work of registered social landlords, such as housing associations, has involved:

i) developing most new socially rented housing;
ii) a funding regime based upon a public–private partnership;
iii) an expanded role as providers of care and support services, including services purchased by health and social services.

5 There has been some revival in private renting – it remains a minority tenure but one that may be used by numerous people with community care needs.

6 'Special needs' housing schemes continue to make an important contribution to those with housing and support needs but they have come under increased criticism for their separation from mainstream provision.

7 Health and social services professionals often have a very narrow view of housing work. The Chartered Institute of Housing defines the following housing management tasks as being core competencies:

i) Lettings, allocations, transfer and nominations
ii) Homelessness and housing advice
iii) Rent collection
iv) Rent arrears management
v) Housing benefits work
vi) Tenant participation and consultation
vii) Repairs reporting, inspection and maintenance systems
viii) Voids management (ie, the management of empty property)
ix) Estate management

8 However, this is the only partial picture of the diversity of work that may be carried out by staff employed by housing providers. Social services and health staff will often need to have contact with care and support staff and with sheltered housing staff, whose work is not reflected in the above list and whose work may be funded from a variety of sources including contracts with social services and health purchasers. Important, yet frequently missing, players in housing/homelessness and community care debates are environmental health officers, because of their pivotal roles in the home improvement grant system, home adaptations and in monitoring housing standards,

including in the private rented sector. Care and Repair and/or Home Improvement Agency staff can also have an important role in advising elderly people and disabled people on improvement and adaptation issues. It also needs to be remembered that housing workers and other staff might be working for the local authority, a registered social landlord (the size and scope of which vary enormously) or a voluntary organisation.

Social services

1 Major changes were brought to the community care system by the 1990 NHS and Community Care Act and associated policy guidance. These included:

  i) social services to be the **lead agency** for all the main community care groups;

  ii) social services to make proper assessment of need and good **care management** the cornerstone of high quality care;

  iii) social services to produce and publish **community care plans** which set out their future purchasing intentions;

  iv) social services to develop its role as an enabling authority;

  v) social services to consider establishing an organisational separation of its **purchasing** activities from its **provider** services (home care, day care, etc);

  vi) social services to take on the key role in the assessment and funding of people seeking **independent sector residential or nursing home care.**

2 Local authorities have been given considerable discretion over how to respond to the challenge of providing services that respond to individual needs and preferences within a mixed economy – organisational arrangements and terminology varies enormously from local authority, and from client group to client group within authorities.

3 At the strategic level, social services authorities have varied in their approaches to community care planning–purchasing. This has seen improved consultation with service users and carers in many authorities. However, the emphasis has tended to be on developing joint agreements with health, particularly in the area of roles and responsibilities with regard to continuing care.

4 One of the main aims of community care policy was to shift the balance between residential and domiciliary care wherever reasonable and practicable. This has been achieved. Sophisticated packages of care and support are now available to people with high support needs in most authorities and many of those might previously have been in some kind of institutional setting. Finding a balance between an effective response to people with high levels of need and continuing to offer assistance to people with lower levels of need is a challenge.

5 There is a growing range of independent sector providers of care at home services in most local authorities, but this remains less developed than for residential or nursing home care, and most local authorities remain major suppliers of home care and other services.

6 The central importance of the housing dimension of community care is increasingly recognised at both the strategic and operational levels.

7 Only a minority of the 300,000 staff employed by social services departments are qualified social workers, and until recently they were much more likely to work in childcare social work than in work with the main community care groups. This is changing and increasingly they are performing key assessment roles in community care with the job titles of care or case manager becoming more common.

8 Other important occupational groups who have traditionally worked for social services include home care organisers and occupational therapists.

9 The 1996 Community Care (Direct Payments) Act, implemented on 1 April 1997, enables social services departments to make direct payments to service users (initially to disabled people under the age of 65) whom it has assessed as needing community care services. This is a power and not a duty, the aim of which is to increase users' independence by giving them more choice and control over the services they receive.

Health

1 A focus on housing and the environment was regarded as important for good health by the 'Health of the Nation' strategy (1992), which advocated a shift of emphasis in the health service from treating illness to addressing the *causes* of ill-health.

2 Far-reaching changes were effected in the healthcare system by the 1990 NHS and Community Care Act. The main change was the purchaser–provider split. This mirrors to some extent the client–contractor split that housing departments have implemented and the purchaser–service provider split often to be found in social services departments. Health Authorities now operate at a strategic level and purchase healthcare services – they no longer manage them. Health Authorities also have public health as well as purchasing functions; they run services such as health promotion and are responsible for the registration of nursing homes. Since April 1996, Health Authorities have replaced the old Family Health Services Authority (FHSA) which used to be responsible for GPs and the District Health Authority (DHA) which was responsible for purchasing healthcare. Health Authorities are responsible for:

i) drawing up strategies and purchasing plans in collaboration with other key agencies including local authorities to meet the needs of their population;
ii) agreeing contracts with the providers of services (NHS trusts; voluntary and private sectors) to meet those needs.

3 In many areas, the role of Health Authorities as purchasers is shared with GP fundholders, who have contracts with trusts for specified services on behalf of their practice populations. This means that a significant part of the healthcare budget lies outside of the direct control of the Health Authority and that partnerships with local authorities can be complicated. Some GPs are working with their local Health Authority to pilot the purchase of a much fuller range of health services and these are known as total purchasing pilot sites. In liaising with Health Authorities, it should be understood that they often cover large geographical areas and relate to several local authorities. Health Authorities need to work closely with all GPs in their area to draw up strategies which reflect the views of primary healthcare teams and their patients. Some Health Authorities have developed 'a locality approach' to purchasing, which may coincide with local authority boundaries.

4 The delivery of services and their management is the responsibility of NHS trusts which are legally separate and independent bodies. Health Authorities agree contracts with the trusts for service provision, set broad quality standards and monitor performance. Among them may be found acute and specialist hospital trusts, community health services trusts, mental health services trusts, learning disability trusts or any combination of these in one trust.

5 Working with health services will be easier if some of the pressures they are working under are understood, such as rising standards and a growing demand for healthcare. A rapidly changing healthcare technology in recent years has led to:

i) higher rates of day surgery not requiring hospital admission;
ii) shorter lengths of inpatient stay in hospital and their earlier discharge from hospital;
iii) many more patients being treated.

6 At the service delivery level, operational joint working exists between individual NHS trusts, local authority departments and the voluntary and independent sectors, but the form it takes may vary from one area to another. You will need to be familiar with these relationships in your local area.

7 Understanding how health professionals in the community are organised is invaluable when working with health-related housing problems (see **Module Two**). The GP and the primary healthcare team have responsibility for individual patients and you will often need to talk to the GP's practice manager, the practice nurse or the GP in a specific practice. Where a person is homeless and does not have a GP, the local hospital casualty department is a first recourse

for emergencies, but for more routine healthcare, the Health Authority should be approached as arrangements do exist so that people without an address can register with a GP. Physical and personal *health*care in the home for highly dependent people is delivered by community nurses employed by the local community health trust but often attached to a local GP surgery. Specialist nurses for incontinence, stoma and terminal care may also be involved. Other kinds of support are generally available from the social services' home care department.

8 Where mental health problems or dementia are concerned, community care and support for individuals in many areas is undertaken by joint health and social services mental health teams, although service users remain the primary responsibility of their GP.

Conclusion

- Joint working is happening.

- Joint working is valuable.

- Joint working is difficult.

- Joint working can be made to work.

- Understanding each other's organisational priorities is an important starting point.

Guide to further reading

Arblaster, L., Conway, J., Foreman, A. and Hawtin, M. (1996) *Asking the impossible?: inter-agency working to address the housing, health and social care needs of people in ordinary housing*, Bristol: The Policy Press. [Recent research based on three case studies in England, a key finding being that professionals have a "widespread lack of conceptual understanding" of the different agencies involved.]

Cowan, D. (ed) (1996) *The Housing Act 1996: a practical guide*, Bristol: Jordans. [A comprehensive and authoritiative account of how the changes introduced by the Act are likely to work in practice.]

Department of Health (1994) *Implementing community care: housing and homelessness*, London: Department of Health. [This study looked at 10 local authorities and concluded that housing was not yet fully integrated into the community care agenda.]

Department of Health (1995) *An introduction to joint commissioning* and *Practical guidance on joint commissioning*, London: Department of Health. [These two documents outline the growing recognition of the importance of joint commissioning by the key statutory agencies.]

Department of Health/Department of the Environment (1997) *Housing and community care: establishing a strategic framework*, London: Department of Health. [The aim of the framework is to ensure the necessary coordination between housing, social services and health at the strategic level.]

Ham, C. (1994) *Management and competition in the new NHS*, Oxford: Redcliffe Medical Press. [A clear assessment of the initial impact of the NHS reforms and a discussion of future options.]

MacFarlane, A. and Laurie, L. (1996) *Demolishing 'special needs': fundamental principles of non-discriminatory housing*, Derby: The British Council of Organisations of Disabled People. [A powerful critique of the tendency to segregate disabled people into 'special needs' housing rather than to integrate them into mainstream provision.]

Meredith, B. (1995) *The community care handbook: the reformed system explained*, London: Age Concern (England). [An excellent handbook and guide to the community care system introduced by the 1990 Act.]

Smith, R., Gaster, L., Harrison, L., Martin, L., Means, R. and Thistlethwaite, P. (1993) *Working together for better community care*, Bristol: SAUS Publications. [Provides a useful summary of the joint working literature and goes on to present six innovative projects and initiatives.]

Watson, L. and Conway, T. (1995) *Homes for independent living: housing and community strategies*, Coventry: Chartered Institute of Housing. [In many ways, this excellent report is complementary to the workbook in that its emphasis is upon joint working at the strategic level.]

[Professional journals, such as *Community Care, Health Services Journal* and *Housing* can be an invaluable source of information.]

Mapping your locality

module two

Introduction

There is no simple answer to 'who does what' in health, housing or social services. Although the main community care, health and housing responsibilities of the statutory agencies are laid out in legislation, authorities at the local level may organise their work differently and take a variety of approaches to discharging these responsibilities. This is before you begin to consider the pivotal contribution of the numerous voluntary and independent sector organisations in any given locality. Thus, the names of organisations, the names of teams and the designations of individual staff are likely to show considerable variation from one locality to another. This means that mapping your locality is a crucial exercise in any attempt to improve joint working at the local level.

Objectives

1 To develop the capacity of staff in health, housing and social services to map each other's organisational functions across the public, private and voluntary sectors.

2 To provide guidance on the range and depth of information required.

3 To offer suggestions as to how the information might be collected together and kept up to date.

- This workbook does *not* propose that all operational staff should map every conceivable agency of relevance to the support, health and housing dimensions of community care in their localities. This would be time consuming and swamp people in unnecessary detail.

- However, team leaders and others responsible for groups of operational staff should have a good grasp of how the main agencies of relevance to their clients are organised locally.

- Care managers, housing workers and other field-level staff should have an awareness of how a wide range of different agencies might be able to contribute to meeting the housing, health and support needs of service users.

Mapping social services

QUESTION 1

Can you distinguish the strategic planning/purchasing/commissioning arm of your local department from its field-level/operational activities?

EXAMPLE

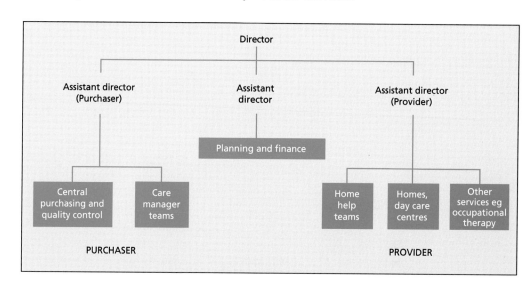

COMMENT

This is a version of a purchaser–provider split in which care managers are seen as the people who 'purchase' services on behalf of the individual client. These services might be from the in-house provider (home care, day care, etc) but they might just as easily be from the voluntary or private sectors.

EXAMPLE

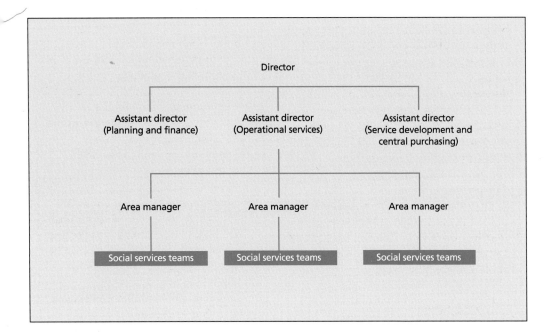

COMMENT

As can be seen, other social services authorities have created a central purchasing unit while assessment and provider roles at the area office level have remained integrated. Such authorities may still have redesignated some staff as care managers but this is less likely than for those operating the previous model.

TASK

Obtain an organisational map of your local social services department which identifies how purchasing and providing activities are organised. Remember: the details of the purchaser–provider system in use is likely to be specific to your authority.

QUESTION 2   **Can you identify who carries out individual assessment and care package coordination roles in your social services authority?**

EXAMPLE

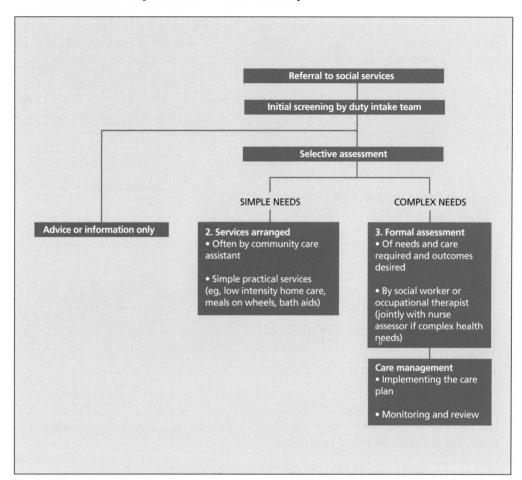

Source: Audit Commission (1996) *Balancing the care equation*, London: HMSO

COMMENT   In this example, initial screening is carried out to determine who requires a more detailed assessment of their needs with a further distinction being made between those with simple and those with complex needs. However, each social services authority will have its own approach to which staff in which teams should assess which applicants. The situation will be equally varied in terms of which staff are responsible for the coordination, monitoring and review of care packages and other support arrangements established as a result of the assessment. Remember that even where social services departments have area officers and teams, some specialist assessment work may well be carried out by teams based at the centre.

TASK   *Identify the assessment and care plan coordination arrangements in your local social services authority which are relevant to the service users that you work with. Remember: some relevant teams, especially in the areas of mental health and learning disabilities, may be inter-disciplinary and cut across health and social services boundaries.*

Do you understand how support services for individuals are 'bought' by social services? To what extent are operational staff involved in purchasing services for their clients?

QUESTION 3

"From 1st April 1995 all budgets for purchasing community care were allocated to social work teams. The Council's directly provided services all now operate on a separate trading basis and are subject to the same arrangements as the independent sector. Social work teams have the freedom to purchase care packages from whichever provider can best meet the needs of the user. No priority is given to in-house services." (Abstract from community care plan)

EXAMPLE

In the above example, the care manager/social worker is able to 'spot' purchase the services which their clients require and they are under no obligation to give priority to services provided in-house. Increasingly, budgets are devolved to such assessment teams. In other authorities the emphasis is more upon the 'block purchase' of services such as day care and home care with the care manager/social worker meeting the needs of people through services which have been pre-bought through a block contract. Some local authorities are developing their own in-house services as a separate trading arm. The 1996 Community Care (Direct Payments) Act means that eligible service users in some localities will be able to 'buy' their own care and support services.

COMMENT

Identify how care services are purchased by your local social services department. At what level is the purchasing budget devolved and what is the role of field-level staff and their team leaders in buying services?

TASK

Do you know the explicit priorities used to decide who qualifies for care management/a full needs assessment/a care package?

QUESTION 4

Order of priority for people living in the community:

EXAMPLE

Older people
Priority 1   To provide appropriate community-based services in order to reduce the requirement for some older people (including those with carers) with complex needs to enter residential or nursing home care on a long-term basis.
Priority 2   To support carers who themselves may need support to enable them to continue caring.
Priority 3   To enhance the quality of life of carers and users.

People with learning disabilities, HIV/AIDS, mental health problems and alcohol/drugs problems, physically and sensory disabled people, and homeless people
Priority 1   To meet the needs of people with complex social care needs who are presently unable to stay in their own homes.
Priority 2(a) To enhance the ability of people to live independently of their families where this is their choice.
Priority 2(b) To rehabilitate people from small-scale hostel-type accommodation into the community where this is their choice and their needs can be met in this way.
Priority 2(c) To support carers who themselves may need support to enable them to continue caring.
Priority 3   To enhance the quality of life of carers and users.

Within existing budgets, it is not expected that it will be possible to purchase services to help people who fall in the Priority 3 categories.

COMMENT

A major source of tension between operational staff from housing and social services can be a lack of understanding of the systems for prioritising those in greatest need which exist in social services.

TASK

Identify the priority systems used by your social services department, concentrating upon their relevance to your own work responsibilities.

Mapping healthcare

QUESTION 1

Are you clear about the role of the Health Authority and GP fundholders as the purchasers of healthcare services and the role of health trusts, voluntary agencies and private agencies as the providers of healthcare?

QUESTION 2

Are you clear how GP fundholders fit into the purchasing of healthcare services?

EXAMPLE

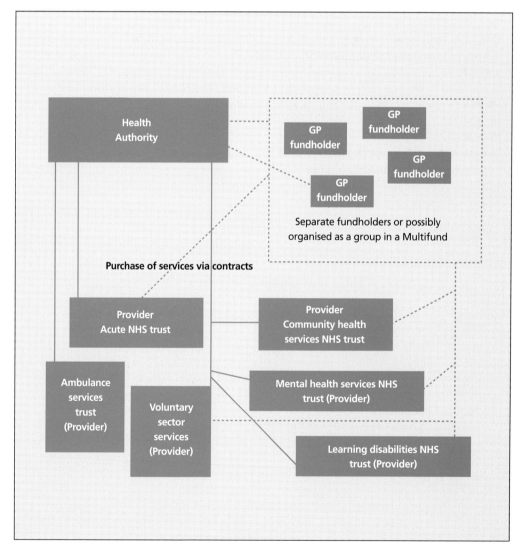

COMMENT

This diagram illustrates the configuration of healthcare purchasers and providers in a typical Health Authority area. However, there will be variations in how healthcare is organised from area to area.

For example:

- in many areas, GP fundholders will have a variety of *individual* contracts with the providers and will be setting a variety of quality requirements and standards;

- in some areas, acute NHS trusts may be organised according to medical specialty and/or according to geography (ie, they cover a designated part of the Health Authority's territory; they may also treat patients from other Health Authorities);

- in many areas, the provision of acute and community health services may be in the hands of one or more dual purpose NHS trusts; this means that the same body is responsible for hospital care as for the delivery of, for example, district nursing services in the home;

- on the other hand, in some areas, community health services are separate from hospital provision; they may also be delivered by general purpose community health trusts or divided between a number of specialist trusts dedicated to a specific client group, such as people with learning disabilities or mental health problems.

Create an organisational map showing who provides hospital, community healthcare, mental health and learning disabilities services in your area. (See also Questions 5 and 6.)

> **TASK**

Do you know what local authorities your local Health Authority covers?

> **QUESTION 3**

How does your local Health Authority organise its purchasing by localities? What are the arrangements for your area?

> **QUESTION 4**

> **EXAMPLE**

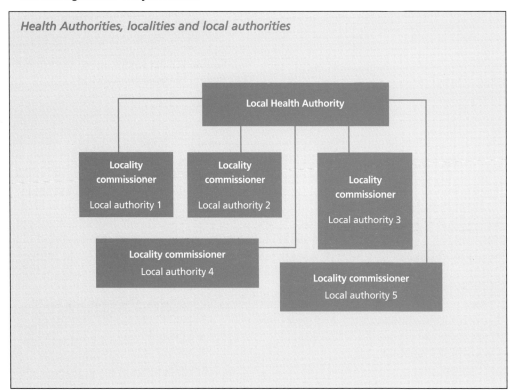

Health Authorities, localities and local authorities

In many areas, the physical territory covered by the Health Authority may be so large that it organises its purchasing activities into localities. These localities often correspond with the area covered by the unitary authorities responsible for social services and housing. Where a large city is concerned, the localities may correspond with urban sub-districts.

> **COMMENT**

TASK

List the local authorities covered by your local Health Authority. Sketch the main purchasing localities of your Health Authority (if it has any).

QUESTION 5

Who are the providers of community health and mental healthcare services in your area?

QUESTION 6

Is there a community mental health team in your area? If not, where are the mental health workers situated?

EXAMPLE

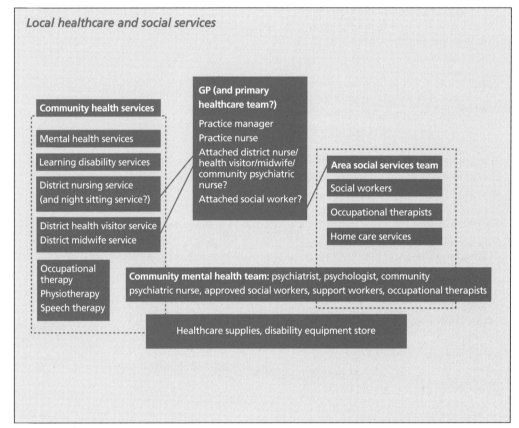

Local healthcare and social services

Community health services

Mental health services

Learning disability services

District nursing service (and night sitting service?)

District health visitor service
District midwife service

Occupational therapy
Physiotherapy
Speech therapy

GP (and primary healthcare team?)

Practice manager
Practice nurse
Attached district nurse/ health visitor/midwife/ community psychiatric nurse?
Attached social worker?

Area social services team

Social workers

Occupational therapists

Home care services

Community mental health team: psychiatrist, psychologist, community psychiatric nurse, approved social workers, support workers, occupational therapists

Healthcare supplies, disability equipment store

COMMENT

This is a simplified organisational map of the interface between primary healthcare, community health services and local social services. Not all GP practices have a full practice team with a practice manager. It is important to note that GP practice areas are defined by where their patients live and so will not usually coincide with any of the boundaries observed by either the health or local authority. A GP's patient lists can contain people from widely varying localities. In the example, healthcare and disability equipment supplies have been shown as a joint service organised across community health services and social services. However, in many areas these will be separate services.

TASK

Make a diagram of the structure and relationships in your area of community health services, primary healthcare and social services.

Mapping housing

Can you profile the main social housing landlords active in your locality and do you understand how to refer applicants to them?

QUESTION 1

EXAMPLE

What is the Portsmouth Housing Register?

The Portsmouth Housing Register is a list of people wishing to rent accommodation or buy a low cost home. To join the list you need only complete this application form. Any of the Partners' own tenants who live within the City boundary and City Council tenants can also use the same form if they wish to transfer/exchange. This form can be used to apply:

• To rent accommodation from the City Council.

• To rent accommodation from registered social landlords.

• To be nominated by the City Council to rent privately owned accommodation.

• To be considered for shared ownership schemes.

Who can be considered

• Anyone aged 16 years or over can be considered.

• You need to complete this form and return it to any of the Partners.

• Completed forms can of course be returned by the applicant direct to the City Council's rehousing section.

Portsmouth Housing Register Partners

Downland Housing Society Ltd
Ektha (Unity) Housing Association
Haig Homes
Housing 21
James Butcher Housing Association
John Grooms Housing Association
Knightstone Housing Association
Portsmouth City Council
Portsmouth Housing Association
Raglan Housing Association Ltd
Samuel Lewis Housing Trust (City and Counties Housing Association Ltd)
Shaftesbury Housing (South West Region)
Sovereign Housing Association
Swathling Housing Society Ltd
Warden Housing Association

COMMENT

Partners to a common register are unlikely to include all the major social landlords since some may decide to retain their own separate application process. Second, it is important to appreciate that common housing registers are still not that numerous. However, the local authority is still likely to have a key role through its own register and associated nomination rights. There may also be opportunities for individuals to apply direct to a variety of other landlords. Remember that a significant number of local authorities have transferred their housing stock to housing associations or to other types of landlord.

TASK

Discover if your housing authority runs a common housing register, and if so, obtain a common application form. Identify up to 10 social landlords of relevance to your own area of work, and how clients might be able to make an application to them.

QUESTION 2

EXAMPLE

What is the spread of specialised housing and support provision in your area?

Local authority/housing association	Bedspaces owned (hostel/ shared housing	Units designed for the elderly	Bedspaces designed for the elderly	Units designed for wheelchair users
Chesterfield				
Anchor Housing Association	36	77	36	1
Carr-Gomm Society Ltd	6	-	-	-
Chesterfield Churches Housing Association Ltd	-	31	-	-
East Midlands Housing Association Ltd	5	36	-	2
Habinteg Housing Association Ltd	11	5	-	9
Hallam Housing Society Ltd	-	14	-	-
Home Housing Association Ltd	2	-	-	-
Housing 21	-	30	-	-
Johnnie Johnson Housing Trust Ltd	-	31	-	-
Northern Counties Housing Association Ltd	95	90	-	2
Salvation Army Housing Association	-	18	-	-
South Yorkshire Housing Association	38	-	-	1
Stonham Housing Association	35	-	-	-
Total	**228**	**332**	**36**	**15**

Source: Housing Corporation (1994) *Housing associations in 1994: local authority breakdown of housing association stock*, London: Housing Corporation, p 103

COMMENT

The range of specialised housing and support schemes is likely to vary enormously from locality to locality. Sometimes the bricks and mortar of the scheme will be the responsibility of a housing association, but care and support workers will be employed by a specialist voluntary organisation. On other occasions, the housing association, the local authority or an independent sector agency may be responsible for all aspects of the scheme. The example provided profiles housing association 'schemes' only, and hence does not include any local authority schemes or specialist voluntary provision run by organisations not registered with the Housing Corporation. It shows the traditional preponderance of schemes for elderly people, but gives little indication about which 'groups' the remaining provision is targeted at. The information provided is generated by a return made by housing associations to the Housing Corporation (form HAR/10/1). Other valuable sources of information include the national database of retirement homes run by the Elderly Accommodation Counsel (Telephone 0181 742 1182).

TASK

Obtain details of the main specialised housing and support schemes of most relevance to your work. Identify their allocation criteria and how to make applications/referrals to them.

Do you understand the network of provision for homeless people in your locality?

QUESTION 3

EXAMPLE

Homelessness path

COMMENT

The homelessness path in each locality will show considerable variation with different assessment routes and different provider agencies being involved. However, nearly all paths will include a combination of statutory and independent sector agencies which cut across housing, social services and health. **Module Three** looks at the different paths individuals will take according to whether they are assessed as 'statutorily' homeless or not.

TASK

Identify the homelessness path in your locality, including key contact names and addresses.

QUESTION 4

Do you understand how to apply for a home adaptation in your locality?

EXAMPLE

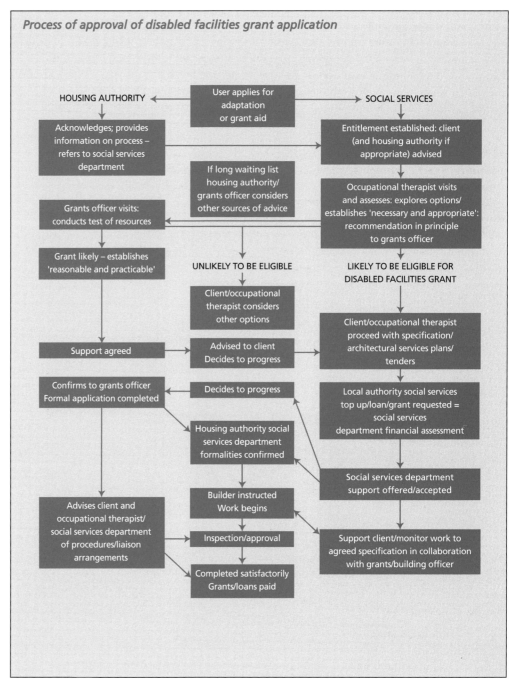

Process of approval of disabled facilities grant application

Module Four looks at issues of home adaptation and the disabled facilities grant. At this stage our aim is to stress the pivotal role of the housing authority. Officers responsible for this grant will normally be designated as environmental health officers, improvement grant officers or housing officers. They will usually be based in the housing department or the environmental health department. In a two-tier authority, they will be based in the district council, while the occupational therapist will usually work for social services in the county council. The example offered illustrates the complexity of the process and the need for housing and social services to work well together in order to minimise time delays.

COMMENT

Identify how to apply for a home adaptation in your locality. Concentrate upon identifying where home adaptation work is based within the housing authority and how occupational therapists are organised within the social services authority. Collect key contact names and addresses.

TASK

Do you understand how the contracting out of housing management services may have affected your local housing department(s)? (NB: Many staff in health and social services relate to more than one housing department.)

QUESTION 5

EXAMPLE

Contracted housing services (run by the Neighbourhood Housing Services):

Tenancy management

Management of communal areas and facilities

Void property management

Responsive repairs

Lettings and allocations

Garages and car parking

Performance and monitoring indicators

General items (tenant participation, equal opportunities, out of hours working, non-standard tenancies etc)

Strategic (client) housing services:

Housing management client function

Housing management contract coordination

Policy development

Liaison with housing associations

Homelessness

Information technology system management and development

Right to Buy and service charges administration

Other house sales initiatives (such as cash incentive schemes)

Allocations of dwellings – this non-tendered function will be devolved to neighbourhoods in the near future

Coordination of sheltered housing

Rent debit control and rent setting

COMMENT

In this example, housing management services have gone out to tender, and the contract has been won by the in-house bidders (Neighbourhood Housing Services). In some authorities, the contract has been won by an external agency (housing association, private sector company, etc) or the authority has delegated their housing management functions to an agency or tenant management organisation. There is some variation in the range of functions retained by housing authorities (ie, the client services).

TASK

Discover if your housing department(s) has completed a contract tendering process. If so, obtain a map of how the contractual services and the strategic (client) services have been allocated.

QUESTION 6

Do you understand how core housing functions are organised by your local housing department(s)? Do these functions continue to include a landlord function, or has all or part of their housing been transferred to a housing association or local housing company?

EXAMPLE

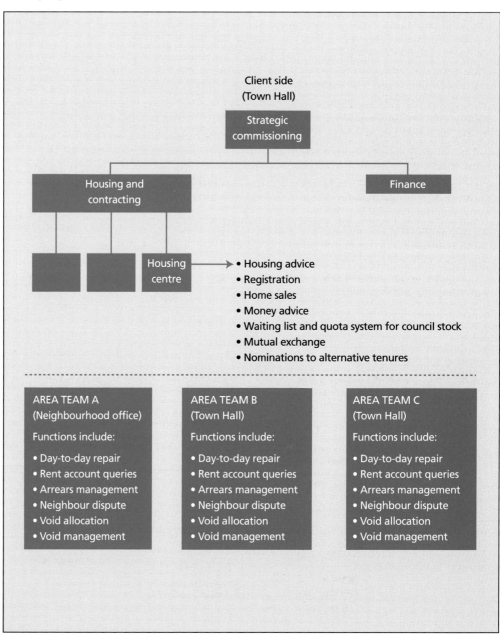

Readers of the workbook require an awareness of contract tendering but most will be in more need of a detailed feel for how specific housing tasks are organised. A key point of likely variation is whether or not there is a structure of area/neighbourhood offices (partly a reflection of the extent to which the local authority remains a major provider of housing). Another is whether the housing management function is separate from lettings/allocations, or if there are 'generic' housing teams who cover both these roles. In the chosen example, the contractor runs three housing teams, two in the Town Hall and one in a neighbourhood office. It is the client side who runs the waiting list applications and computer processing functions, creating a list which can be accessed by the area teams in order to identify potential applicants for their voids. Thus, the contractor makes the letting, but from a list managed by the client.

Obtain an organisational map of your local housing department(s). Identify the main sections and their housing functions.

Expanding your map

In trying to understand health, housing and social services, it is important to take a broad view when mapping relevant agencies. The range of agencies and organisations who may be able to meet some of the housing and support needs of individuals is vast, as can be seen from our table on expanding your map (below). **Remember:** the aim is *not* to try and know everything but to collect mapping information of relevance to your roles and responsibilities. But in doing this remember that one of the aims of the community care changes was to enable service users "to achieve their full potential" (Department of Health [1989] *Caring for people: community care in the next decade and beyond*, London: HMSO, p 3). This requires professionals to work together to respond to quality of life issues and to consider service users within their broad social support networks.

Of particular relevance is the need for field-level staff to be aware of the full range of advice and advocacy services which are available locally. This is crucial because the statutory agencies may only be able to respond to those they assess as in priority need. It is important to be aware of other agencies which may be able to offer additional support and advice in addition to that provided by the statutory agencies.

Extending the map

Organisations of service users/disabled people/carers	Advice and advocacy agencies	Providers of care and support services	Other sources of support
These might include: Coalitions of disabled people Survivors Speak Out People First Care forums Young carers groups etc	*These might include:* Citizens Advice Bureau Shelter Money Advice Project Welfare Rights Project Disability Advice Centre (perhaps run by disabled people) Advocacy Project (perhaps run by disabled people) etc	*These might include:* Age Concern MIND Mencap Crossroads Private domiciliary agencies Centres for Integrated Living (perhaps run by disabled people) etc	*These might include:* Religious organisations Libraries Leisure clubs Stroke clubs Lunch clubs Drop in centres etc

TASK   *Identify those organisations of most relevance to your own work, including contact names and addresses. Pay particular attention to local advice and advocacy services.*

Possible short cuts: many Councils of Voluntary Service or their equivalent produce excellent directories of local organisations. Check whether or not your local social services department keeps its own directory.

Mapping and joint training

The task set out in this Module may appear tedious and time consuming. However, the task can also be an excellent focus for joint training. Participants from different agencies could bring their owns maps to training events, and relate this to how each saw their roles and responsibilities. This means that **mapping can be enjoyable**, and part of an **educational process** based on **dialogue** rather than just the filing away of information.

Maps get out of date

However, organisations are constantly changing in terms of structures, priorities and personnel. Maps become out of date unless they are updated on a regular basis. First-line managers and field-level staff *must* update their maps, but again this can be linked to training events and team meetings so that the implications of these changes for the future joint working can be discussed and drawn out.

This Module has made numerous suggestions about information that operational staff need to collect about each other's agencies. It is important that this is pulled together by teams and/or individuals into a resource file. This needs to include not only organisational maps but also detailed information on contact names, address and telephone numbers.

Because of the variety of backgrounds and information requirements of the readers of the workbook, it is not possible to offer a single model for capturing all of this information in the most appropriate and accessible form. A number of options are offered throughout the workbook in terms of how to develop contact lists and service directories. The example offered in this Module is therefore made for illustrative purposes and readers should feel able to adapt to meet their own purposes.

EXAMPLE

Resource file entry

Name of organisation _____   Opening hours _____

Address _____   What service provided _____

Fax _____   Referral/procedure _____

Contact person _____

Conclusion

- Mapping your locality as proposed will greatly increase the effectiveness of your joint working by providing a much clearer picture of other key agencies.

- Take care to concentrate upon collecting what is of most relevance to you, including contact names and addresses.

- Update your map at regular intervals.

Assessment and care management

module three

Introduction

Department of Health guidance defines care management as "the process of tailoring services to individual needs". There is considerable variety in the way care management is organised. Social services departments deal with a large number of wide-ranging referrals for assistance. One of the main aims of care management is to ensure that, when the assessment decision is that services should be provided, they are well planned and coordinated. This might involve working closely with other agencies. The tasks of care management (see below) will be carried out by a number of different staff in social services. Often the allocation of a specific care manager, on a long-term basis, will only occur when individuals require intensive help because of complex and changing needs.

Objectives

1 To develop housing workers' understanding of assessment and care management systems.

2 To develop social services staff's understanding of the assessment and provider roles of housing agencies.

3 To facilitate improved inter-agency working across the public, private and voluntary sectors.

4 To develop the confidence of staff in risk assessment.

Assessment and care management

It is easy to assume that there is consensus about what we mean by assessment and care management. Department of Health guidance to social services authorities has defined care management as having seven core tasks:

1 **Publishing information:** making public the needs for which assistance is offered and the arrangement and resources for meeting those needs.

2 **Determining the type of assessment:** deciding on the best way to carry out an assessment and who needs to be involved.

3 **Assessing need:** looking at a person's problems and circumstances, in partnership with them and their families and carers, and deciding, in the light of agency policies and priorities, how to assist them.

4 **Care planning:** negotiating the most appropriate ways of achieving the objectives identified by the assessment of need and incorporating them into an individual care plan.

5 **Implementation of care plan:** securing the necessary resources or services.

6 **Monitoring:** supporting and monitoring the delivery of the care plan on a continuing basis.

7 **Reviewing:** reassessing needs and the service outcomes with a view to revising the care plan at specified intervals.

(Department of Health/Social Services Inspectorate, 1991)

The objective of a community care assessment is to determine the best way to help the individual and "every effort should be made to offer flexible services which can enable individuals and carers to make choices" (Department of Health, [1989] *Caring for people: community care: the next decade and beyond*, p 9).

Factors to be taken into account in an assessment

Biographical details

Age, family circumstances, religion and ethnic origin.

Self-perceived needs

Self-care

How well the person can carry out basic tasks such as eating, dressing or bathing; how well they can get around.

Physical health

Checking whether a request for social care arises from a health need which could be improved.

Mental health

Checking to see whether a mental health need has developed unnoticed or unreported. The assessor will have to judge when it is appropriate to consult a health worker, such as the GP or a community psychiatric nurse.

Use of medicines

Checking to see if there are problems in taking essential medicines, and whether a pharmacist, GP or nurse should be involved.

Abilities, attitudes and lifestyle

Checking the person's situation in relation to their own expectations.

Race and culture

Appreciating racial and cultural diversity when identifying individual needs and how to deal with them.

Personal history

Making sure that the effects of past events – perhaps a bereavement – are fully taken into account in assessing present needs.

Needs of carers

Carers should always be aware of their entitlement to be involved and to be consulted (within the constraints of confidentiality). It should never be assumed that carers will have the same views about needs and care as the person being assessed – the assessor will have to weigh up the different views. Carers who are providing substantial and regular care have had a *right* to request an assessment of their ability to care or to continue to care since the implementation of the 1995 Carers (Recognition of Services) Act.

Social network and support

What other help is available, apart from immediate carers?

Care services

What services are already being received, and how appropriate are they now?

Housing

Housing authorities and/or other providers (such as housing associations) should always be involved in the assessment if there may be a housing need.

Transport

Some needs may arise because of lack of suitable transport – for instance, to get to the shops.

Risk

The assessor will have to weigh up these risks, with emphasis given to the person's entitlement to self-determination and independence (always bearing in mind that person's capacity to take informed decisions).

Finance

Assessors will be urged to make sure that the person being assessed and their carer(s) receive all the benefits to which they are entitled. Assessors will also have to test the means of the person being assessed, to see how much, if anything, they should pay towards the cost of care.

Source: based upon B. Meredith (1995) *The community care handbook*, London: Age Concern, pp 82-3

What is the Care Programme Approach?

Some users of the workbook will have heard of the Care Programme Approach (CPA) and wonder if it is different from care management. CPA was introduced in 1991 to provide a framework for the support of people with mental health problems outside hospital. It has four elements:

- systematic arrangements for assessing the health and social needs of people accepted by the specialist psychiatric services;

- the formulation of a care plan which addresses the identified health and social care needs;

- the appointment of a key worker to keep in close touch with the patient and monitor care;

- regular review, and if need be, agreed changes to the care plan.

Overall, CPA places a high emphasis upon involving users and carers, and upon multi-disciplinary assessment.

Although Social Services Departments have responsibility for care management, and Health Authorities for the CPA, **the principles underlying the two processes are the same**.... If properly implemented multi-disciplinary assessment will ensure that the duty to make a community care assessment is fully discharged as part of the CPA, and there should not be a need for separate assessments. (Department of Health [1995] p 15)

Importance of joint working with housing

There is recognition in both care management and care programming of the need to work with housing staff. However, initial research on the implementation of the community care reforms suggested that this was not happening on a systematic basis. For example, the Department of Health (1994) report on *Implementing caring for people: housing and homelessness* devoted a chapter to 'Individual assessment' and found that "links between community care and housing assessment processes varied, and formal triggers for joint assessment were rare" (p 23). The report concluded that housing agencies needed to be brought more centrally into the assessment and care management process.

The Code of Guidance on Parts VI and VII of the Housing Act 1996 recognises the need for housing staff to work closely with care management and care programme arrangements. Housing staff are advised that effective liaison is needed where housing applicants may have care needs and that they should help to deliver the most appropriate solution to the housing support and care needs of such individuals.

Such concern about joint working between housing and social services at the operational level is based upon a belief that its success is important from the point of view of both partners. At its crudest, the reasons why this is so can be broken down in the following way:

1 Why bring in housing?

i) The care manager is not sure of their client's housing needs and hence wishes to access a specialist housing needs assessment (eg, of the damp in the house, of their tenancy rights, of their entitlement to a home improvement grant, of whether they are homeless as defined by housing legislation, of whether their housing is inappropriate, etc).

ii) The care manager wishes to access housing or housing services for their client (eg, a council house, a housing association property, a housing and support scheme, a home adaptation, a private sector tenancy, etc).

iii) The care manager needs to work with the housing professional to address issues of rent arrears, housing repair and maintenance, conflict with neighbours, etc.

2 Why bring in social services?

i) The housing professional is not sure of the care and support needs of their client and hence wishes to access a specialist community care assessment.

ii) The housing professional wishes to access services provided or funded by social services such as home care, respite care or a place in a residential or nursing home.

iii) The housing professional needs to work with the care manager to sort out their tenant's existing care package, to address issues relating to the distressing behaviour of neighbours known to social services, to assess whether the housing situation is exacerbating their social care needs, etc.

The above suggests that it might be more helpful to think in terms of the complementary assessment roles of both housing and social services staff rather than just in terms of joint assessments. It also underlines that joint working between housing and social services raises issues throughout the care management process and not just in relation to assessment.

Key questions and issues

1 Assessment by care managers and other social services staff: what housing questions should be asked during assessment as a matter of routine?

2 Assessment by housing workers: what community care questions should be asked during assessment as a matter of routine?

3 Complementary assessments: how can we develop trigger questions on assessment forms which are seen as helpful and, hence, used by housing and welfare professionals? How can we become clear about who is the lead assessor for each individual and what assessment input is required from each party? How should issues of confidentiality be addressed?

4 Allocation decisions: what influence should each agency have on the allocation of accommodation and/or care services provided by or funded by the other agency? How can the eligibility criteria of agencies including registered social landlords be developed so that they enhance the possibilities of coherent inter-agency responses (eg, accommodation panels, etc)?

5 Involving housing workers in the monitoring and review of care packages: are housing workers involved fully in the review of housing and support packages?

6 Requests for a reassessment: how should requests for a reassessment from housing staff be responded to by social services?

Asking the right questions

1) Care management and housing questions

As a matter of routine, social services staff need to explore with individuals whether an effective response to their needs requires action relating to their present housing situation. Social services staff should be sensitive to the possibility that housing *is* a problem, even if this is not raised initially during assessment. This is because some people may not be aware of the different ways in which they might be helped.

Both social services and housing staff need to agree with service users the answers to the following types of questions (based on Arnold et al, 1994):

• How suitable is the accommodation in which you are currently living? Does your housing (or lack of it) in any way contribute to your difficulties?

- What regular support or help do you currently get? Is it enough? How do you manage?

- Would adaptations to your housing reduce your difficulties, or your dependence?

- Would a different place to live reduce your difficulties or dependence? What kind of place? Would you contemplate such a move? What support or help, if any, would you still need?

(See Hounslow example opposite.)

Where clients identify their housing as a problem, the care manager needs to ask straightforward questions about the person's present housing situation (tenure, mobility problems in the house, mortgage arrears, etc) and their perception of their housing requirements (home adaptation, transfer to ground floor accommodation, etc). For homeless people and other vulnerable tenants, appropriate questions might include:

- How many times have you had to move in the last year?

- In what circumstances did you lose your last home?

- What types of accommodation have you been living in recently (hostel, friend's floor etc)?

- Are you paying for this 'accommodation'?

The collection of housing information enables social services staff to make a decision about whether they are able to resolve or respond without a more specialist housing assessment.

The knowledge of the care manager on housing issues may often be fairly basic, so that a housing 'assessor' can be more perceptive on the diagnoses of the housing problem and more creative about offering solutions. Also, the care manager may wish to access housing resources on behalf of their client via

someone with a detailed grasp of local housing policies. Housing authorities have the central role in this, especially in view of their new duty under the 1996 Housing Act to secure the provision of advice services. However, there is still no single housing 'door' in most localities and so care managers may still need an understanding of local housing agencies and referral options.

As indicated in **Module One**, housing professionals have a variety of housing jobs and hence the focus of the housing assessment will vary according to what this is. However, among the questions housing professionals could tackle for social services staff would be:

- **Appropriateness?** Size, location, access to community services; effects on health (dampness, heating, state of repair); privacy (shared facilities); accessibility (to and within the accommodation).

- **Affordability?** Rent arrears; mortgage arrears; housing benefit assessment.

- **Personal security?** Security of tenure; racial harassment; conflict with neighbours; noise.

Housing professionals will often be able to prioritise clients on the basis of the above assessment. Reasons for prioritisation include:

- health or medical needs;

- social reasons (housing and social services need an agreement on vulnerability definitions);

- accessibility/suitability;

- overcrowding/underuse.

Local housing policies on how to prioritise and the extent to which there should be a response to those with social reasons for wanting a move will vary enormously, reflecting views of members, stock availability, etc. There is often a mismatch between what housing is wanted and what is available, so that second best options may have to be negotiated.

Hounslow: community care – general assessment of need

1. Are you a council tenant   Owner-occupier   Private tenant   Boarder/lodger
                                        ☐   ☐   ☐

    Other, please specify: _____

2. Which floor do you live on?
    please specify _____

                                                                    Yes   No

3. Do you use a lift to get to the floor where your home is?   ☐   ☐

4. Do you use stairs to get to your home?   ☐   ☐

5. Has your home been altered/adapted for your physical needs?   ☐   ☐
    If you have answered 'yes' to Question 5, please list below
    the works that have been done or any that have been arranged
    for the future _____
    _____
    _____

6. How do you heat your home?   Central heating   ☐
                                            Gas fire   ☐
                                            Electric heater   ☐
                                            Coal/log fire   ☐
                                            Calor gas   ☐
                                            Paraffin   ☐
                                            Other _____
                                            (please specify)
                                                                    Yes   No

7. Do you have an indoor lavatory?   ☐   ☐

8. Do you share any of the following with another family?
                                            Bathroom   ☐   ☐
                                            Toilet   ☐   ☐
                                            Kitchen   ☐   ☐

9. Does your home have   Dampness   ☐   ☐
                                      Condensation   ☐   ☐
                                      Pests (eg, mice,   ☐   ☐
                                      cockroaches)   ☐   ☐
                                      Draughty floors   ☐   ☐
                                      Draughty windows   ☐   ☐

10. Do you have problems with   Access   ☐   ☐
                                      Social aspects   ☐   ☐
    Please explain _____
    _____

Social services staff need to have the following knowledge and skills:

• awareness of how housing is organised locally, what their priorities are and what housing agencies might realistically be likely to provide (NB: housing authorities must provide free copies of a summary of their housing allocation schemes);

• this awareness to include an understanding of both options for homeless people and vulnerable tenants, together with options for those seeking advice on home improvement and/or adaptation;

• knowledge of how to make appropriate referrals to housing agencies;

• knowledge of how to respond appropriately to referrals from housing agencies;

• awareness of alternative sources of help and advice (advocacy groups, organisations of service users/disabled people, specialist voluntary agencies, etc);

• commitment to work in partnership with service users and their advocates.

Social services staff cannot demand a response from housing agencies but they can encourage a (re)assessment to be made where they have concerns about their clients' housing situation.

2) Housing workers and community care questions
Housing workers equally need to think through what questions about care and support to ask their tenants/clients and under what circumstances. Housing staff need to keep in mind a number of 'trigger' questions which suggest someone may have care and support needs. These include

• Does this individual have a clear need for specific social services?

• Is this individual vulnerable? (including for health and medical reasons?)

• Is this individual 'at risk' of losing their home/failing to find accommodation without care or support?

• Is this individual experiencing a breakdown of social support?

• Is this individual a source of anxiety to neighbours?

---

5. Care and support at current address

5.1   Do you already have (✓ below any that apply)

Social worker	☐	Community nurse	☐
Key worker	☐	Occupational therapist	☐
Probation officer	☐	Home carer	☐
Community psychiatric nurse	☐	Other	☐

If you do have any of the above, please give name of person (and office or organisation address, including telephone number where applicable) as we may wish to contact them.

_____

5.2   Do you feel you need any additional form of care and support to enable you to stay where you are until you are moved   Yes ☐   No ☐
If YES - what eg: Home care, community alarm, aids and adaptations, eg: grab rails, stairlift _____

Would you like an assessment to see how this care and support could be provided
                                                                    Yes ☐   No ☐
Please give the name(s) and date(s) of birth of the person(s) who need(s) this care and support:
Name:_____   DOB: _____
Name :_____   DOB: _____

Source: Portsmouth's common housing register application form

Housing staff need to have the following skills and knowledge in such situations:

- awareness of how social services and health are organised locally, what their priorities are and what they might realistically be likely to provide;

- knowledge of how to make appropriate referrals to health and social services, including information required by social services;

- knowledge of signs of possible dementia and when to seek further advice;

- ability to recognise possible signs of crisis and vulnerability;

- alternative sources of help and advice (advocacy groups, organisations of service users/disabled people, specialist voluntary agencies, etc);

- a commitment to work in partnership with the tenant, housing applicant or their advocate.

Housing staff cannot demand that health and social services provide services, but they can encourage a specialist assessment to be made where they have concerns about a client or tenant.

3) Towards complementary assessments

By asking the right initial questions, and by developing agreed trigger questions and shared assessment forms, housing and social services staff can begin to develop a complementary approach to assessment. The majority of social services authorities and housing authorities are beginning to develop joint assessment forms such as the Dorset one outlined below. However, a fully complementary approach to assessment requires housing and social services staff to develop confidence about when to trigger such joint assessment procedures.

Dorset Social Services

Housing – social services joint assessment form (Abstract)

Housing needs and support (please ✓ appropriate box)
Is the applicant capable of managing a tenancy independently?   Yes ☐   No ☐
Please give details: _____

Is the applicant capable of managing a tenancy with support?   Yes ☐   No ☐
Give details: _____

Has a full social services care management assessment been carried out?   Yes ☐   No ☐

What support does the applicant need? _____

Interval at which this will be reviewed (eg, every six months) _____

What support will be provided by:
Social services _____
Housing _____
Other agencies (please state name of agencies) _____

Does the applicant have specific housing requirements/needs: Yes ☐   No ☐
If Yes, give details: _____

Action/Outcome:
Action agreed: _____ By whom: _____ By date: _____

Assessment and homeless people

The focus of the first half of this Module was on how to draw housing and housing staff more fully into care management and/or care programming. The starting point of this section is the large numbers of both homeless people and vulnerable tenants who have support needs, who have difficulty accessing health or social services or whose needs will not always be severe enough to ensure that they are deemed as being in priority need from the point of view of social services. Such individuals are likely to require health and social services, but only some will have allocated key workers or care managers.

Local housing authorities have a duty to secure the provision of advice and information about homelessness and the prevention of homelessness to people in their area. Authorities can choose whether to provide this service themselves or whether to support other advice agencies. Through this mechanism, or alongside it, the voluntary sector is likely to continue to play an important role in advising people who are homeless or who are threatened with homelessness.

Local housing authorities also have specific accommodation responsibilities to those homeless people who are homeless, in priority need and who have no suitable alternative accommodation available to them. Priority need can come from having dependent children, being pregnant or being the victim of fire, flood or other disaster, or being vulnerable due to old age, mental illness, learning disability, physical impairment or major health problem. Many people in the 'vulnerable' category are likely to have both housing and support needs. However, allocation of a local authority secure tenancy or nomination for a registered social landlord assured tenancy must be via obtaining sufficient priority on the housing register.

> **Shelter Lincolnshire's freephone advice line**
> Shelter Lincolnshire is a small independent advice centre based in Sleaford, a town of about 10,000 inhabitants, but provides an advice service for the whole of Lincolnshire. Because the centre covers a large area, much of its advice work is carried out over the telephone. Some people drop in to the centre or telephone directly, but a large proportion (about 70% of cases) are referred by other agencies. The centre is involved in a project called Advice Links, which provides a freephone advice line through local CABx, and refers housing problems to Shelter Lincolnshire. Case workers can then contact clients by telephone. (Grant, 1996, p 31)

Voluntary agencies have long argued that homeless people with support needs require a coordinated response from a wide range of agencies and yet this often fails to happen. This is partly because they work with large numbers of people who are either on the margins of homelessness as defined by the law or who are assessed by the statutory agencies as not vulnerable under the homeless legislation or not eligible for community care services.

Duty to provide housing advice
Housing Act 1996
• Housing advice services to be available to everyone in the area.
• Advice and assistance to the non-priority and intentionally homeless.
• Prevention of homelessness by helping people keep existing accommodation.
• Provision of advice and assistance in place of duty to accommodate where suitable alternative accommodation is available in the local authority's district.

Source: Grant (1996) p 9

Homeless and other vulnerable people are likely to face numerous obstacles to obtaining an appropriate response to their needs:

- they may not understand assessment routes;

- they may have difficulty accessing mainstream services;

- they may have trouble registering with GPs;

- they may have multiple needs which cut across the eligibility criteria of different agencies;

- they may be highly mobile;

- they may get passed around from agency to agency;

- they may lack advocacy skills or someone to advocate on their behalf;

- they may lack information on how to access their benefit entitlement;

- they may lack money.

Ways forward

1 **Understanding services for homeless people at the local level:** running throughout this workbook has been an emphasis upon understanding the organisational structures and priorities of other agencies so that this information can be used to the advantage of service users. Health and social services staff who have homeless clients or who advise homeless people need:

- an understanding of homelessness law as amended by the 1996 Housing Act;

- an understanding of local services for homeless and other people in vulnerable housing situations (eg, advice services, local hostel provision, etc).

As repeatedly emphasised, local services will show great variation from local authority to local authority. How does your locality compare with the example given in **Module Two**?

2 **Understanding health and social services provision at the local level:** housing and other staff working in services for homeless and other vulnerably housed people need to understand how local health and social services are organised, how to make a referral to them and what their priorities are. (See **Module Two**.)

3 **Retaining contact:** a major challenge in this area of work is that people can be difficult to engage and maintain contact with, and so they can easily become 'lost'. For example, prisoners with severe mental health problems require both housing and mental health services on release, and this may require housing staff to liaise with the probation service as well as health and social services. However, any housing move (eg, a change of hostel or a move to more permanent housing) may require a transfer between mental health teams. A failure to achieve this can easily lead to a breakdown in the housing arrangement, and hence a possible drift into homelessness. Advocacy can be especially important for people who struggle to work with formal systems.

4 **Finding a route into assessment:** a key difficulty faced by many homeless people is that they struggle to even get themselves into the assessment system for consideration of their housing, health and support needs. Their needs are only partially assessed or they slip through the net altogether. One key to avoiding this happening is the development of a strong housing advice function (see Reading example). There is a growing recognition of the need to develop innovative outreach and multi-agency projects to improve routes into assessment for homeless people. For example 'Help and Advice for People in Housing Crisis' is a multi-agency project in Bristol (the Hub Project), which provides a single point of access to a number of organisations able to provide help and advice to people in housing crisis. Equally crucial can be good housing advice.

Reading Borough Council's advice service

At Reading Borough Council the advice service is the first point of call for most housing-related enquiries. When people come to reception looking for new accommodation or with a housing problem, they are usually given an appointment with a housing adviser at a later date, or asked to call in to one of the service's drop-in sessions. If the problem is urgent, they are seen immediately.

On interviewing people presenting as homeless, advisers assess whether they appear to be owed a duty under homelessness legislation. If they seem to be homeless and could be in priority need, they are given advice on their rights and referred to the homelessness section for an assessment interview. Otherwise the adviser gives the client information on other housing such as local hostels and night shelters, and goes through longer term options for finding accommodation, including possibilities in the private rented sector and details of the council's rent deposit scheme.

For cases of disrepair, arrears, harassment, unlawful eviction or other problems, the advice services give help and support to tenants and advice on legal remedies.

As well as reactive casework, the housing advice service works to increase the availability and affordability of privately rented housing. This includes producing Good Landlord Guides, a deposit guarantee scheme, fast tracking for housing benefit, a private sector housing forum and a county court surgery. It also provides training on housing rights and options to staff working for other parts of the council, local agencies and landlords.

Source: Grant (1996) p 38

Hub – an inter-agency initiative

Bristol Cyrenians are the 'front of house' team who welcome people to the Hub. They offer general advice on welfare benefits, housing debt and homelessness issues and can make referral to the other agencies in the Hub.

Shelter provides a specialist advice and advocacy service for any problems relating to housing or welfare benefits.

Avon Health link workers enable people to access appropriate healthcare services. They also make referrals to statutory and voluntary agencies such as the Council on Alcohol and Drugs, the Bristol Drugs Project and social services.

Social services staff provide short-term support and put clients in touch with people who can provide support for longer term need.

The employment service has details of job vacancies and can give general employment or careers advice.

Careers Service West holds information about education opportunities and training.

Homelessness caseworkers of the housing department are able to assess individuals' eligibility for immediate assistance in line with the law on homelessness.

The Deposit Bond Scheme aims to help people gain access to accommodation in the private rented sector. The deposit bond worker is able to issue a guarantee or bond to landlords enabling people to obtain tenancies.

The Benefits Agency provides advice and information across the whole range of social security and assists where necessary with the completion of claim forms.

5 Complementary assessments between housing and social services: the broad principles of joint working and complementary assessments are laid out earlier in this Module.

6 Developing care plans and care programmes: the first half of this Module looked at this in some detail. Three points need to be added:

- voluntary organisations can play a key role in developing care plans and care programmes in partnership with service users and the statutory services;

- care plans and care programmes must consider issues of access to primary healthcare (see **Module Five** for detailed discussion);

- homeless people should be encouraged to consider accommodation which combines housing and support only if it meets their needs and never just because there are vacancies in local schemes.

Assessment and support for vulnerable tenants

Housing agencies are increasingly concerned about the large numbers of tenants they house who are vulnerable but who receive only limited if any direct support from health and social services. For example, a tenant may have alcohol problems which results in their experiencing problems in many aspects of their life.

Such tenants in both the socially rented and the private rented sectors may be vulnerable to eviction and subsequent homelessness because of such factors as rent arrears, unkempt homes and complaints from neighbours. Professionals working with such tenants should be encouraged to draw upon good practice in assessment and care management in order to resolve problems and to support the maintenance of tenancies. Below are two examples of how local authorities have attempted to respond positively to this challenge.

Supporting vulnerable tenants (Example One)

The housing and social services department in the London Borough of Haringey has established a small housing support team of two workers to help vulnerable tenants experiencing problems in maintaining their tenancies. Referrals to the team are made solely by the borough's area and neighbourhood office housing managers. At the initial visits, a standard checklist assessment is used covering benefit entitlement, repair needs, contact with GPs etc. Follow-up work depends on the outcome of the initial assessment and can involve referral to social work teams for a full assessment. The housing support team bridges the gap between services through its client-centred approach. It has successfully accessed support for the 'non-coping' single tenant from doctors, nurses, social workers, housing workers, benefit agency staff and voluntary sector workers.

The staff of the housing support team are funded through the housing revenue account and this represents a creative use of resources since 70% of cases have serious rent arrears at the first visit, a situation addressed primarily through ensuring benefit entitlement is claimed in the future.

Supporting vulnerable tenants (Example Two)

Eastbourne Borough Council have a special needs housing officer funded from Health Authority joint finance money and from contributions from housing and social services. The worker is employed by the housing department, but spends part of her time with social services. Her brief is to assist people who have housing difficulties and support needs. She acts as an assessor for housing needs, identifying the right housing situation, but also helping the client access the support services needed to make that accommodation work.

A flexible use of housing and support options

Those working with people with housing, care and support needs must have a clear grasp of available provision and options, and the capacity to use these creatively to address the needs and aspirations of service users. Where gaps are identified, this information needs to be fed back by field-level staff and their team managers to those with strategic purchasing responsibilities. The balance of options will vary from locality to locality but included in the workbook below are a small number of creative attempts at finding solutions to the housing and support requirements of individuals.

For most people, the solution to their housing and support needs will be to help people to say put in their existing accommodation. However, for those such as homeless people, some frail elderly people and young disabled people wishing to leave the parental home, an appropriate housing and support solution will involve finding 'new' accommodation. In these circumstances, agreement between housing and social services on eligibility criteria for sheltered housing, for other types of housing and support schemes and for the delivery of care and support is crucial. For example, it is crucial that there is agreement across the different agencies about the roles and responsibilities of sheltered housing staff. An increasingly common approach to tackling this challenge is through the establishment of inter-agency allocation panels, often backed up by joint agreements and protocols on eligibility criteria.

Floating support and homeless people

The Housing Services Agency (HSA) in London manages both hostel and self-contained accommodation for single homeless people. The latter includes flats from two housing associations' general needs stock, which are offered to people who are assessed as needing intensive ... support, of varying levels for varying period of time. HSA offers four different options concerning the provision (or not) of furniture and payment of bills. Each tenant's needs are assessed and an individual plan, including a timetable of targets, is drawn up and agreed between the housing manager and the tenant. The housing manager's job description includes ... the following tasks:

- to identify tenants' support needs and to refer to external bodies for appropriate support to enable them to benefit from their housing ie welfare rights, debt counselling, liaising with DSS/Housing Benefit Department and, where necessary, to act as their advocate when dealing with outside bodies;

- to ensure maximum take-up benefits for tenants through liaising with Welfare Rights Worker, DSS/Housing Benefit Department;

- to assist tenants with debt problems, ie debt counselling and money advice;

- to keep up to date with any relevant changes in benefit regulations/welfare rights;

- to take responsibility for clients by providing them with support and counselling in personal welfare matters.

These tasks are in addition to the standard housing management tasks of collecting rents, dealing with rent arrears, repairs, inspection of voids, tenant participation, and so on. The housing manager is also involved in the allocation and letting of properties.

Source: Morris (1995)

Floating support and people with HIV/AIDS
Strutton Housing Association aims to provide "self-contained accommodation for people with HIV and AIDS in housing need in London, managed in a way which enables them to lead full and independent lives...". Strutton specifies detailed and high quality design criteria and since 1991 has sought to develop all new units using 100% Housing Association Grant and SNMA [Special Needs Management Allowance]. However, the ... support provided is 'floating' in the sense that it responds to changes in tenants' need for support. While the notional staff/tenant ratio is 1:20, "Strutton estimate that at any one time some Strutton tenants will require an input equivalent to a ratio of 1:5, whilst others will be getting by quite happily with an input equivalent to 1:100."

Source: Morris (1995)

People with learning disabilities
KeyRing is a charity providing supported living opportunities for people with learning disabilities in nine London boroughs and one neighbouring county. It sets up low level support systems, known as networks. A community living worker, who lives in the vicinity, helps people to manage their tenancy, obtain access to other services, find mutual support and generally become integrated into the local community. Wherever possible, the worker seeks to link tenants with other local people, under a principle of fostering good neighbourliness.

All the tenants served by the KeyRing have mild or moderate learning disabilities and are fairly independent, but would not cope easily on their own. They come from the parental home, residential homes (as a move toward more independence), living on their own and not coping and, in some cases, sleeping rough. The target age range is 18-60 but most are in their 30s.

The flats in which people live are independent of one another and the people are seen as ordinary tenants. Most are local authority properties, but some belong to housing associations. The community living workers are mostly part-time and unpaid, receiving free rent and related bills paid in recompense for their work. They have a lengthy induction period and regular supervision. KeyRing intends to involve tenants on interview panels for new workers in other networks. Each network is also independently evaluated annually.

Source: Mental Health Foundation (1996) p 51

People with mental health problems from the African Caribbean community
Makonnen House is a housing and support project in Manchester for men of African Caribbean origin who have mental health needs. It was developed as a partnership between Creative Support (a voluntary organisation) and North British Housing Association to meet an identified need for high levels of support for African Caribbean men who are represented in disproportionately high numbers with the mental health system. The project offers the following:

• two adjacent houses with 24-hour staffing – one offering a high level of support with seven bedrooms and en-suite bathrooms; the second house offers a lower level of support and houses four tenants;

• support for 6-18 months to enable tenants to become confident to live more independently;

• African Caribbean staff team with knowledge of local community;

• an emphasis on enabling service users to identify their own needs and preferences.

Sheltered housing is changing: the emerging role of the warden

Sheltered housing is changing!
Sheltered housing was originally intended for fit active older people. Wardens were employed as 'Good Neighbours' and received little training. But demographic trends and community care have led to a much older and frailer population living in sheltered housing.

The role of the warden is therefore evolving. Most housing organisations have reviewed the service provided and have put into place new job titles and descriptions, training, procedures, guidance and management systems. (The new job titles include: scheme manager, resident manager, estate manager, sheltered housing officer). Many wardens have undertaken the one year National Wardens Course/Certificate in Supported Housing.

Wardens are key professionals who:
• are required by their employers to monitor well-being by maintaining usually daily contact with the older people living in their schemes;
• building up a trusting and unique relationship with tenants over months or years;
• are aware of the total range of statutory private, voluntary and family support that a tenant receives.

Wardens are:
• housing professionals with responsibilities towards buildings and tenants;
• managers of sheltered housing, not hands-on carers;
• there to enable older people to live independently with privacy, dignity, security and fulfilment;
• able to assist with communication solutions due to sensory impairment, language or illness (including dementia);
• able to supplement busy care managers' or hospital staffs' assessments with properly recorded observations made over the preceding days or weeks;
• trained to encourage older people to ask for support, to respect refusal of offers of help and to give information on the availability of and access to services;
• ideally placed, with tenants' agreement, to contribute to assessments and the monitoring of care packages.

Social services and healthcare professionals are encouraged to:
• talk to the sheltered housing managers and wardens in their areas to agree collaborative working arrangements and to clarify respective policies, eg, on medication, lifting, emergency cover, referral, monitoring, etc;
• devise policies and practices which involve wardens in multi-disciplinary assessments, case conferences and hospital discharge meetings where tenants consent; this would be in accordance with the spirit and intentions of community care legislation and funding arrangements;
• invite wardens and their managers to team meetings to explain their role, its potential and boundaries;
• to ensure that older people living in sheltered housing and wardens have copies of complaints procedures and hospital discharge procedures and that their use is encouraged.

Source: Based on leaflet funded by the Housing Corporation and supported by 34 housing organisations

Meeting the needs of people with autism
Autism is a disorder which affects skills needed for social integration and communication.
A large Victorian semi-detached house in Sunderland is now home for seven autistic
people. The two flats are Housing 21's first registered care home, in partnership with
European Services for people with autism. Referrals come from social services
departments, Health Authorities and other agencies from as far afield as North Yorkshire
and Strathclyde.

Source: Based on article in *Inside Housing*, 6 September 1996

Monitoring and review

It is crucial that housing and support
arrangements are monitored and
reviewed with the service user and any
advocate they may have (see review
example.)

- Are they satisfied with the housing and support they are receiving?
- Is the plan/care programme working to their satisfaction?
- Do they wish to move on to perhaps a more independent style of living?

Review in the context of care management/care programming
Rita Evans has a severe learning difficulty and is profoundly deaf; she is 46 years old. She
had lived in two hospitals for 30 years. In the mid-1980s she moved out under a
resettlement programme and was housed by Friendship Care Choices with 20 other people
in an inner-city district of Birmingham.

The accommodation was ahead of its time, being designed in small domestic units and
part of a general housing development in the area by Friendship Housing. Rita settled in
well at first, sharing with three other people. She grew and developed many new personal
skills and aspirations and chose many of the things that were important to her, like the
colour of the decoration in her room, the furniture she used, where she wanted to go, and
the staff who supported her. As she developed she became dissatisfied living in a group
setting, but because she has no verbal communication she was unable to say so. She
demonstrated her feelings by getting frustrated and angry. The other people who lived in
the house found her equally difficult to live with.

Her key worker, together with the home leader and with the assistance of the local
psychologist, explored with Rita why she seemed so unhappy. Getting to the crux of the
matter was not a straightforward process. Visits, photographs, smiles, tears and even
anger were all part of the process, but it became apparent that Rita wanted a home of her
own rather than to share with others. Rita's disposition became more positive as she
embarked upon flat hunting, and she was over the moon when she found one.

A partnership agreement with health and social services was drawn up, under which
Friendship Care Choices provides the 24 hours a day support Rita needs to be able to live
independently in a flat provided by another housing association. This was an innovative
care package made up of support workers, some of whom she already knew, good
neighbours and other volunteers.

Rita is happy – she has many good friends and neighbours, her own flat and her own
tenancy, and supporters she can rely on. Friendship Care Choices has been supporting
Rita for the last eight years, and today she has a service we can all be proud of, one shaped
by herself. She lives in her own home: the support she receives enables her to do so. For
the first time Rita is in charge of her own life. Her journey from hospital to residential
care to her own home has been a success.

What is essential is that housing staff should be drawn more centrally into the monitoring and review process. There needs to be clear agreement about when housing needs to be a partner. Over and above regular reviews, any agency involved in providing housing or support must be seen as having the right to involve other agencies when circumstances change or a crisis occurs. Equally, regular review meetings need to be robust with a willingness to 'close' cases where ongoing inter-agency involvement is no longer required in order to achieve the objectives of the care plan.

Developing joint procedures and protocols

Not only are shared assessment forms, agreed trigger questions and accommodation panels becoming more common between housing and social services but there is also a trend towards joint procedures and protocols. These commonly address issues of reassessment, review and monitoring as well as initial assessment. Some are partial in terms of the client 'groups' or the types of housing covered while others attempt to be more comprehensive (see boxed Salford example below).

Such developments are an excellent sign of a genuine commitment to improved joint working. However, it is *crucial* that these are developed in a way which is consistent with the principles laid out in **Module One.**

Do (✓)

• Develop procedure and protocols in partnership with organisations of service users and carers.

• Develop these in partnership with operational staff from housing, social services and other relevant agencies.

• Use these in partnership with individuals receiving or requiring services as a mechanism for meeting their housing and support needs.

• Make sure procedures which claim to be comprehensive cover all housing options and situations (owner-occupation, private renting and social renting) and not just housing and support schemes such as sheltered accommodation.

• Encourage the creative use of local agencies to meet the needs of individuals in partnership with the main statutory agencies.

City of Salford: housing and social services departments joint referral procedure – contents

1.	Priority rehousing scheme	2.	Children Act rehousing
3.	Allocation of adapted properties	4.	Disabled facilities grant
5.	Allocation of sheltered housing	6.	Mobile warden services
7.	Medical assessment points and procedures	8.	Clients with HIV or AIDS infection
9.	Homelessness and community care	10.	Clients with learning disabilities
11.	Clients with mental health problems	12.	Notification of impending eviction
13.	Monitoring	14.	Good practice
15.	Two-way referrals	16.	Establishing networks
17.	Further developments	18.	Arbitration
19.	Contact list	20.	Hostels list
21.	Referral list	22.	Case agreement
23.	Monitoring form		

Don't (X)

- Develop procedures and protocols without consulting both organisations of service users and carers and operational staff from partner agencies.

- Use these in a way which excludes individuals from the central role in deciding appropriate responses to their needs and preferences.

- Use these to exchange confidential information on a routine basis with no agreement from service users.

- Use these as a service-driven device to coerce people with housing and support needs into difficult-to-let housing and support schemes (hostels, sheltered housing, etc).

Exchanging information about individuals

Joint assessments, allocation panels and joint protocols all require the exchange of information about individuals if they are to work to the advantage of service users. The increased willingness of professionals from health, housing and social services to do this is a very positive development. However, it is vital that issues of *confidentiality* are thought through. Professionals often claim that personal information is only passed on to other agencies on a 'need to know' basis. What should this mean in practice?

There may be occasions ... where the sharing of such information is sensible and can expedite the allocation process ... although authorities will wish to preserve confidentiality and supply information only on a need to know 'basis'. (Department of the Environment/Department of Health [1996] *Code of Guidance in Parts V1 and V11 of the Housing Act 1996)*

The most detailed thinking about good practice and confidentiality has occurred with regard to people with severe mental health problems. The advice of *Building bridges* (Department of Health, 1995) was as follows:

- the patients should be made aware that, in order that for NHS and local authority social services (or other services, such as probation, housing or voluntary agencies) to plan and provide effective care, personal information may need to pass between them; in most cases this could be covered as part of the usual care planning process;

- information passed on should be restricted to that in which the recipient has a legitimate interest; the recipient should not transmit it to a third party unless the latter is entitled to it or the patient either has explicitly consented or is aware that information needs to be passed on to enable care to be coordinated properly;

- there may be particular circumstances in which disclosure of information is required by statute or court order or exceptionally, in the absence of consent, can be justified in the public interest (eg, in certain circumstances this may be so if someone has a history of violence); disclosures based on public interest involve weighing that interest against the duty of confidence in the *particular* set of circumstances;

- it is important to share the right amount of information with those who need to know; for example, telling staff that an individual is violent is likely to be less helpful than detailing in what circumstances they are likely to be violent and how such situations can be avoided;

- decisions on disclosure of information should be based on the facts that are available, not on supposition or rumour.

Remember: individuals want you to exchange relevant information in order that they can get an appropriate inter-agency response to their needs, but are concerned that this exchange should be carried out in a responsible and professional manner.

Risk assessment

Joint assessments, allocation panels and agreed protocols on case review and reassessment are all centrally involved in risk assessment. Risk takes many forms and includes:

- **Risk from health conditions** (eg, diabetes or epilepsy).

- **Risk from environmental hazards** (eg, use of gas cooker by someone with dementia).

- **Risk of social rejection from neighbours** (eg, the lifestyle or behaviour of the person may lead to rejection and even hostility from neighbours).

- **Risk of exploitation from others** (eg, someone with a learning disability moving from the parental home to an independent flat).

- **Risk of self-harm** (eg, concerns about the possibility of someone attempting suicide).

- **Risk of violence to others** (eg, the person has psychiatric episodes where they may be violent towards other people).

- **Risk of self-neglect** (eg, the person has periods of depression which results in them not cleaning the house, cooking for themselves, etc).

Good inter-agency working sees professionals sharing information between themselves and with service users and carers in order to make an assessment of such risk from a perspective which is committed to maximising the capacity of the individual to retain self-determination. This is an important aspect of weighing up care plan options and for responding to review situations where a care plan is 'failing'. Operational procedures on risk assessment should be part of joint working arrangements between housing, health and social services. Risk assessment will need to include housing staff as partners in the assessment of risk and in agreeing strategies for managing that risk where they have knowledge of the individual or the risk is relevant to their housing circumstances. The development of joint protocols and procedures between housing and social services show that housing is being brought into joint approaches to risk assessment.

When carrying out a risk assessment it is crucial to **involve staff with day-to-day contact** with the individual so that they are committed to the decisions taken and are aware of what support is available from their agencies. For example, it is crucial to involve the warden of a sheltered housing scheme when one of their residents has dementia and a care review is being held.

Violence and risk assessment

In a minority of cases, the possibility of violence to others will sometimes be a factor in a risk assessment, and this issue tends to have a high profile in many joint procedures and protocols. This is to be encouraged so long as care is taken to:

- discourage staff from making unjustified assumptions based on the mental health, physical well-being or past history of the tenant causing concern;

- discourage staff from making unwarranted connections between an episode of violence and a known history of mental health problems (most people with mental health problems are not violent – only a minority become violent because of their mental health problems);

- discourage staff from passing on unnecessary information in an effort to reassure and build up trust.

In order to avoid these pitfalls, operational staff need access to the following:

- **Clear operational policies and training on violence:** staff need advice, guidance and training on how to minimise the likelihood of encountering dangerous and violent situations, and how to react if they nevertheless find themselves in such a situation. This is *not* a policy relating to working with certain people with particular mental health problems but a more general recognition that most field-level staff will encounter potentially violent clients on occasions.

- **Training on mental health, dementia etc:** housing and other staff need basic information and guidance in order to give them confidence. We would especially recommend *Mental health care: a guide for housing workers* by Thompson et al (1995).

Mental health checklist

1 Do you know how to contact your local:

- Mental health team?
- Social services department?
- Neighbourhood beat officer?
- Mental health advocacy centre?
- Users/self-help group?
- Mental health charity centres?
- Citizens Advice Bureau?

Do you have a contact name for each?

2 Do you know what to do if:

- You suspect someone has a mental health problem, and needs help?

- Someone you suspect has mental health problems is not paying their rent, or causing other housing administration difficulties?

- Neighbours complain about the behaviour of a person with mental health problems?

- There is a violent incident involving someone in mental distress in your neighbourhood office, or on the estate?

3 Have you received interview and communication skills training?

4 Do you have access to mental health literature, and someone to discuss mental health problems with?

5 Do you have a referrals and assessment procedure with your local mental health teams?

6 Do you know how to set up a service delivery package with other community services?

Source: Thompson et al (1995)

Guide to further reading

Anderson, I., Kemp, P. and Quilgars, D. (1993) *Single homeless people: a report for the Department of the Environment*, London: HMSO. [Reports on a survey of 2,000 single homeless people.]

Arnold, P., Page, D., Bochel, H. and Broadhurst, S. (1994) *Community care: the housing dimension*, York: Joseph Rowntree Foundation. [Looks at the vital area of how housing needs might be identified and incorporated into community care assessments.]

Bines, W. (1994) *The health of homeless people*, University of York: Centre for Housing Policy. [Reports on a survey of 2,000 single homeless people.]

Department of Health (1995) *Building bridges: a guide to arrangements for inter-agency working for the care and protection of severely mentally ill people*, London: Department of Health.

Department of Health/Social Services Inspectorate (1991) *Care management and assessment: practitioners' guide*, London: Department of Health. [An accessible account of what is meant by care management in the terms of the community care changes brought in by the 1990 Act.]

Edwards, A. (1996) 'Is care management being implemented?', *Community Care Management and Planning*, August.

Goss, S. (1994) *The housing aspects of AIDS and HIV infection: a manual for housing professionals*, London: HMSO. *The housing aspects of AIDS and HIV infection: a manual for health and social care professionals*, London: HMSO. [These two reports offer detailed guidance on inter-agency working with regard to meeting the housing needs of people with AIDS and HIV infection. Many of the checklists, trigger questions and suggested approaches are also highly relevant to other 'groups'.]

Grant, C. (1996) *Housing advice services: a good practice guide*, Coventry: Chartered Institute of Housing. [This guide looks at statutory duties to provide advice, housing advice strategies and the role of advice in preventing homelessness.]

Health Advisory Service (1995) *A place in mind: commissioning and providing mental health services for people who are homeless*, London: HMSO. [Covers operational as well as strategic issues.]

Hudson, J., Watson, L. and Allan, G. (1996) *Moving obstacles: housing choices and community care*, Bristol: The Policy Press. [This study looks at the extent to which the housing moves made by people requiring extra support or care services reflect their individual choices and preferences.]

Jones, A. (1995) *The numbers game*, Oxford: Anchor Publications. [Looks at a range of issues relating to sheltered housing and black and minority ethnic elders.]

Kitwood, T., Buckland, S. and Petre, T. (1995) *Brighter futures*, Oxford: Anchor Publications. [This includes a look at how elderly people with dementia in sheltered housing are responded to by the tenants and by wardens, and makes suggestions as to how this situation might be improved.]

Lart, R. (1997) *Crossing boundaries: accessing community mental health services for prisoners on release*, Bristol: The Policy Press. [Documents how the Wessex Project identified prisoners with mental health problems in need of services in the community and used the Care Programme Approach to coordinate packages of care for their release.]

Mental Health Foundation (1996) *Building expectations: opportunities and services for people with a learning disability*, London: Mental Health Foundation. [This report is the product of a committee of enquiry chaired by

Dame Gillian Wagner and includes a very useful chapter on housing.]

Morris, J. (1995) *Housing and floating support: a review*, York: Joseph Rowntree Foundation and York Publishing Services. [A review of the strengths and weaknesses of existing floating support schemes and a consideration of how effective they are in helping people live independent lives.]

Riseborough, M. (1995) *Opening up the resources of sheltered housing to the wider community*, Oxford: Anchor Publications. [A practical guide to making sheltered housing a base for the delivery of responsive community care services and social activities.]

Simmons, K. (1995) *My home, my life: innovative ideas on housing and support*, London: Values into Action. [Offers a wide range of innovative responses to the housing and support needs of people with learning disabilities.]

Thompson, K. et al (1995) *Mental health care: a guide for housing workers*, London: Mental Health Foundation. [As suggested by the title, this guide is targeted at the needs of housing workers and includes coverage of the legislation, how mental health services are organised, the importance of joint working and common questions.]

Home adaptation and home improvement

module four

Objectives

1 To provide a checklist of repair and adaptation issues which are likely to affect health and the provision of health and social care.

2 To clarify what help is available from housing authorities and providers to improve poor housing conditions.

3 To explain and clarify the responsibilities of health, social services and housing in providing adaptations to housing for disabled people.

4 To provide examples and ideas for cooperative working between the operational staff of housing, health and social services to achieve warm, safe, comfortable and well-adapted housing.

Context

Warm, safe, comfortable and well-adapted housing can make a great contribution to community care, just as poor or unsuitable housing can prevent or undermine it. This presents a problem for health and social care professionals, because older and disabled people are more likely than other groups to live in housing in poor repair and to suffer illness or accident because of it. There are remedies for poor or disabling housing, however, and this is a sphere where cooperation between health, housing and social services can be especially fruitful when trying to help individuals. Some exciting projects are underway and the potential for other creative partnerships is considerable.

Checklist of repair or adaptation issues relevant to community care

The table on home improvement and adaptation lists housing factors which health and social services staff may wish to consider when they visit people in their home. The column on the right provides key word suggestions about the kinds of help that might be available to tackle the problem. Further details concerning these key words are given in the sections below on home improvement and adaptation.

For many housing problems there are several different possible sources of help, but budgets may exist for one solution and not for another. Health and social services staff will need to enlist the help of housing staff to advise them on what will be the most effective response for their service users at any given time.

Care and Repair, England have a housing assessment form which combines home improvement and adaptation issues. An adapted version is to be found in their training pack *Home for good* in the section on 'Points to look for in the home environment' in the form of two loose-leaf sheets which can be taken out and photocopied (Bradford, Mares and Wilkins [1994]).

Home improvement
Statutory responsibilities and powers

The owner is the person responsible for keeping the property in reasonable condition, although some tenancy agreements may specify certain items for which the tenant is responsible. Section 605 of the 1985 Housing Act (as amended by Paragraph 85 of Schedule 9 of the 1989 Local Government and Housing Act) required local authorities to consider the condition of housing in their areas at least once a year. Where

Home improvement and adaptation: possible sources of help

Housing issue	Tick here	Possible source of help
Are all the rooms the person uses (including bathroom and bedroom) warm and free from mould or damp, so they are not at risk from cold/damp related illness?		Landlord (if tenant), Renovation grant (RG), Home Repair Assistance (HRA), Disabled facilities grant (DFG), Agenda 21, Healthy Cities, Home Energy, Efficiency Scheme grants (HEES), Community Care grant, Home Improvement Agency (HIA)
Is the property physically safe – or are there dangerous stairs, worn carpets, slippery floors, suspect gas fires or electrical wiring or other dangers? Have smoke detectors been fitted?		DFG, RG, HRA, action by an environmental health officer (EHO), HIA
For services users with challenging behaviour are there other safety factors which ought to be considered, such as safety glass, high fencing, window locks etc?		DFG, HRA
Is there a hot water supply, bathroom and indoor WC?		RG, HRA (discretionary), DFG (mandatory), HIA
Can the service user reach to open windows, unplug sockets, change bulbs, etc?		HRA, DFG, handy person scheme, HIA
Is the need for major repairs (eg, roof or windows) causing physical ill health or mental stress?		Landlord (if tenant), RG, HIA, action by EHO
Is the service user worried about possible burglary or attack? Can they open the door safely to carers or to casual callers?		DFG, HRA, HIA, police services, other security schemes
If someone in the house has impaired mobility, have they got access into and around the building so that they can use all the facilities and be as independent as their impairment allows?		Landlord, DFG, HRA, HIA
If there is sensory impairment, would enhanced lighting or adaptations for hearing loss make for greater safety and independence?		DFG, HRA, HIA
Can carers (whether professional or voluntary) perform tasks (especially lifting) safely and without risk of injury to themselves or the disabled person?		DFG, HRA, HIA
Is the patient/service user looking for help that will enable them to stay in their own home? What are their priorities?		HIA or Disabled Person's Housing Service (DPHS) might help householder consider the options in a well-informed way
Is upkeep of the house or garden causing depression or anxiety?		Handy person schemes
Could a housing provider/authority help overcome any of these problems?		Council housing department, EHO, housing association, HIA, DPHS

housing authorities, normally through environmental health officers, find a property to be unfit for human habitation (ie, unfit in respect of the housing fitness standard set out in Section 604 [as amended] of the 1985 Housing Act) they must decide the "most satisfactory course of action". If they conclude that formal fitness enforcement action should be taken, the options open to them are to require that the property be repaired; or that it should be demolished; or to defer action. In the case of deferred action the housing authority is required to review a deferred action notice within two years and at the time of review to consider again the "most satisfactory course of action". (For further details, see Department of the Environment Circular 17/96, in particular, Annexes A and B.)

Repair/renovation: action that can be taken

Health or social services staff who discover housing which is prejudicial to the health and well-being of their patient or service user or carer have various courses of action:

- persuade the owner to improve or repair (this applies to council and housing association properties as well as to owner-occupiers and private landlords);

- ask an environmental health officer to inspect the property and whether they can issue a notice ordering the landlord to make the property 'fit' (ie, safe and in reasonable repair);

- in extreme cases, an environmental health officer can put a 'closing order' on a property, so that no one can live there until certain repairs are carried out; councils may offer rehousing to tenants of private landlords in such cases;

- suggest the occupier applies for a grant (see details in table on repair and renovation, and below) – and seek the advice of the housing grants department about this;

- ensure that the householder understands the timetables, upset and cost that may well be involved in improvement and repair and also the fact that in some cases triggering action by an environmental health officer may lead to the individual having to move temporarily or permanently;

- refer the householder to a home improvement agency, if there is one (see the section on other possible sources of help, below).

Repair/renovation – grants and other sources of help

The table on repair and renovation shows the main forms of grant that exist for both renovation and repair, and who is eligible to apply for them, though grant aid may not be the only source of help or action.

1 **Renovation grants (RGs):** the 1989 Local Government and Housing Act gave to owner-occupiers of unfit properties the right to a mandatory grant (subject to a means test) to make their property fit. The 1996 Housing Grants, Construction and Regeneration Act, most of which came into force on 17 December 1996, replaced the mandatory renovation grant with provisions which are broader in scope than those of the 1989 Act but are to be given entirely at the discretion of the local housing authority.

2 **Home Repair Assistance (HRA):** this is a grant which replaced 'Minor Works Assistance' (called 'assistance' because it can be given in cash or materials). 'Minor Works' assistance, however, was chiefly restricted to people over 60. HRA is available to anyone (except council tenants) in receipt of one of a range of means tested benefits (see table). With the exception of council tenants it is also available to all elderly, disabled or infirm applicants over 18, and to people caring for such a person, whether they are in receipt of benefit

or not. There is no additional means test, nor any requirement for social services assessment, and as the grant may be used for repair, improvement or adaptation it is likely to be useful for a wide range of service users.

3 **Other housing grants:** housing grants also exist for work to the common parts of shared buildings (eg, blocks of flats) and to houses in multiple occupation (HMO). Called respectively 'Common Parts' grants and 'HMO' grants, both are discretionary under the 1996 Housing Grants, Construction and Regeneration Act, but will often be relevant to the users of community care services.

4 **Other grants**

i) **Home Energy Efficiency Scheme (HEES) grant:** this offers help with insulation, draughtproofing and other energy saving measures. Grants are available to anyone on Income Support and also (although at a lower rate) to people over 60 who are not on Income Support. The 1995 Home Energy Conservation Act, which came into force on 1 April 1996, has established energy conservation authorities based on housing authorities and given them the duty to prepare reports on energy efficiency measures. It is worth enquiring whether there are any local initiatives.

ii) **Community Care grant:** this can be used to help make housing more suitable for those leaving institutional care or who would otherwise be at risk of entering it. Ask for form SF300 from the Department of Social Security for details of eligibility criteria.

Other possible sources of help

• **Home Improvement Agencies (HIAs):** the most common of these are (Anchor) 'Staying Put' and 'Care and Repair' projects but other names are used. They can be linked to housing associations or small independent organisations while some local authorities run their own in-house agencies. HIAs were originally set up to help older people tackle problems of disrepair and poor housing and they also play an increasing role in helping secure home adaptation for disabled people. Typically staffed by three people (a care worker, a surveyor and an administrative assistant), they offer the kind of one-stop practical help which is highly valued by service users. They will help the householder consider what work to do, apply for grant aid if needed, and choose a builder. They will supervise the work and also help with benefit checks and any other follow-up measures. They work in close cooperation with local authorities and may receive funding from the housing authority, registered social landlords, the social services authority, the Department of the Environment, Transport and the Regions and possibly the Health Authority. Additional income is generated through charging modest fees (which are themselves grant aidable) on grant work. HIAs are now serving a wider range of service users, and not just older people. They have a national coordinating body, **Care and Repair, England,** who can be contacted by telephone for information and advice on 0115 979 9091.

• **Agenda 21:** these are projects relating to the environment (including energy conservation) which followed the World Conference on the Environment in Rio. Local areas have evolved their own projects, but it is worth enquiring whether there are any schemes which would help deal with heating issues.

Repair and renovation

A. Name of grant	B. Purposes	C. Who eligible?	D. Terms	E. Conditions
Renovation Grant	To make fit To put into good repair To provide insulation, heating system, safe internal arrangement, means of escape from fire, and radon remedial measures. There is also power for the Secretary of State to specify other measures	Owner-occupiers or tenants of private landlords	Discretionary No limits specified Test of resources prescribed by the Secretary of State	Property to be at least 10 years old Applicant must have owned or (if tenant) lived for at least 3 years in the property (except grant for fire escape – or if property is in a Renewal Area or other exceptions). Grant to be repaid if house sold within 5 years of date of grant approval (with exemption in certain circumstances). Local authority has discretion to disregard all these conditions
Home Repair Assistance	To carry out works of repair, improvement or adaptation Help may be in the form of cash grant, or provision of materials, or both	Owner-occupiers, all tenants except council tenants and people with the right to occupy for at least 5 years, who, in each case are aged 18 or over and in receipt of a means tested benefit. Includes owners or tenants of houseboats or mobile homes if certain conditions are met Any owner or non-council tenant who is elderly, disabled or infirm – they do not have to be on benefits Any owner or non-council tenant – they do not have to be on benefits – who needs the work in order to care for someone who is elderly, disabled or infirm	Discretionary. Applicant or partner must be in receipt of Income Support, Family Credit, Housing Benefit, Council Tax Benefit or Disability Working Allowance unless they are elderly, disabled or infirm, or the grant is to care for someone who is elderly, disabled or infirm No further means test Maximum $2,000 per grant or $4,000 in 3-year period (may be altered by the Secretary of State)	Applicant must have lived in property for at least 3 years unless assistance is for fire escape, or to enable elderly, disabled or infirm person to be cared for or property is in a Renewal Area

Note: This table is provided only as a guide. Full details need to be checked in the 1996 Housing, Grants, Construction and Regeneration Act, Part 1 and in subsequent Circulars.

- **Healthy Cities** (often called after the name of the local authority, eg, 'Healthy Birmingham'): again these are locally planned schemes, but might have a programme relating to housing conditions.

- **Disabled Persons Housing Services (DPHS):** although not so numerous as HIAs, DPHSs offer a wide range of housing services to disabled people of all ages and their number is growing. The national body can be contacted by telephone on 01937 588580 and will offer advice about whether there is a DPHS in your area, or help if you want to consider starting one.

- **Handy person schemes:** these are not as numerous as perhaps they should be. They normally carry out minor repairs, maintenance in house or garden, and measures to enhance security, warmth, comfort and safety – usually for older people. They may be employed by council housing departments, HIAs or a range of voluntary groups.

- **More ideas:** Bradford, Mares and Wilkins' *Home for good: making homes fit for community care* (1994) has excellent lists on sources of help or information on problems of warmth, repair, security etc at the end of each 'Practitioner's guide' section.

Good practice: many HIA staff have received training and a HEA/City and Guilds certificate in providing energy advice to householders.
The NEA (a national energy efficiency charity) will supply information about this and other schemes. Telephone 0191 261 5677.

Repair and adaptation

Networking: contacts for help with housing repairs and improvements for social services and health staff

	Name	Telephone
Principal landlord area manager(s)		
Principal landlord repairs		
Principal landlord emergency repairs		
Environmental health officer responsible for enforcement action on housing		
Housing grants officer		
HEES project		
Key housing association contacts		
Home Improvement Agency		
Disabled Persons Housing Service		
Agenda 21		
Handy person scheme		
Any other local projects _____		
_____		
_____		

Repair and adaptation

Networking: contacts for help with support services for housing staff or environmental health officers, if they feel that the practical building work needs to be backed up with a package of support from health or social services

	Name	Telephone
Social services care management team leader		
Social services team manager for physical disabilities and/or elderly people		
Social services home care manager		
Social services other		
Social services occupational therapy manager		
Community health services (for district nurses)		
Locality manager		
GP practice manager		
Community psychiatric nurses		
Health (other key people)		
Voluntary groups		

Repair and renovation
Networking: important information for social services/health staff to discover

What is the strategic approach of the local housing authority to giving Renovation Grants?

• What are the criteria?
• How long would an applicant wait?
• What are the priority categories?

Is the local housing authority giving Home Repair Assistance? If so:

• What are the criteria?
• How long would an applicant wait?
• Are there priority/urgent categories?

Is the council housing department, or any local housing association, willing to rehouse owner-occupiers or private tenants whose homes are in very bad condition? Who would you contact about this?

If there is a Home Improvement Agency? What range of work does it do? What catchment area does it serve and is there a long waiting list?

Adaptation

Statutory responsibilities and powers

- The primary duty to see that the needs of disabled people for housing adaptations are met lies with social services authorities, under the requirements of the 1970 Chronically Sick and Disabled Persons Act, reiterated by subsequent legislation, including the 1989 Children Act and the 1990 NHS and Community Care Act.

- Since 1990, however, part of this duty has been covered by housing authorities through the requirement on them to give mandatory disabled facilities grants to those who meet the criteria. This duty has been reiterated in the 1996 Housing Grants, Construction and Regeneration Act. Any housing authority which is not itself a social services authority has a duty to consult social services. The items for which grant must be given, if other criteria are met, are listed on p 68.

- For all other disabled people, including those who cannot afford their contribution to disabled facilities grant, the duties of the social services under the 1970 Act remain.

- Housing authorities *may* also award discretionary disabled facilities grants or Home Repairs Assistance grants (but these are also discretionary) for adaptation.

- Health and social services employers have duties of care towards their employees in respect of lifting patients in their home, including a duty to have the risk assessed by an appropriately qualified person.

- Department of Health advice requires hospitals to consider the issue of suitability of a patient's home, including adaptations, as part of the pre-discharge procedure.

Although not a legal duty, some social landlords may fund adaptations for their tenants from their own resources. It is worthwhile checking the position locally.

In the sphere of adaptations, even more than that of renovation, the need for cooperation is paramount, with the centrality of the user and the fact that it is their home, never forgotten.

Role of the social services authority to assist with adaptations: Department of the Environment guidance on disabled facilities grants

5 Social services authorities' responsibilities under Section 2 of the Chronically Sick and Disabled Persons Act 1970 to make arrangements for home adaptations are not affected by the grants legislation. Where an application for DFG has been made, those authorities may be called upon to meet this duty in two ways:

(a) where the assessed needs of a disabled person exceeds the scope for provision by the housing authority under section 23 of the 1996 Act; and

(b) where an applicant for DFG *has difficulty in meeting his assessed contribution* determined by the means test and seeks financial assistance from the authority.

6 In such cases, where the social services authority determine that the need has been established, *it remains their duty to assist....* Social services authorities may also consider using their powers under section 17 of the Health and Social Services and Social Security Adjudication's Act 1983 to charge for their services where appropriate.

From Paragraphs 5 and 6 of key guidance on social services departments' responsibility from Department of the Environment Circular 17/96 Annex I (prepared in consultation with the Department of Health). [Emphasis added.]

Mandatory disabled facilities grant: 1996 Housing Grants, Construction and Regeneration Act

The purposes for which an application for a disabled facilities grant must be approved, are the following:

a) facilitating access by the disabled occupant to and from the dwelling or the building in which the dwelling or, as the case may be, flat is situated;

b) making the dwelling or building safe for the disabled occupant and other persons residing with him;

c) facilitating access by the disabled occupant to a room used or usable as the principal family room;

d) facilitating access by the disabled occupant to, or providing for the disabled occupant, a room used or usable for sleeping;

e) facilitating access by the disabled occupant to, or providing for the disabled occupant, a room in which there is a lavatory, or facilitating the use by the disabled occupant of such a facility;

f) facilitating access by the disabled occupant to, or providing for the disabled occupant, a room in which there is a bath or shower (or both), or facilitating the use by the disabled occupant of such a facility;

g) facilitating access by the disabled occupant to, or providing for the disabled occupant, a room in which there is a wash handbasin, or facilitating the use by the disabled occupant of such a facility;

h) facilitating the preparation and cooking of food by the disabled occupant;

i) improving any heating system in the dwelling to meet the needs of the disabled occupant or, if there is no existing heating system in the dwelling or any such system is unsuitable for use by the disabled occupant, providing a heating system suitable to meet his needs;

j) facilitating the use by the disabled occupant of a source of power, light or heat by altering the position of one or more means of access to or control of that source or by providing additional means of control;

k) facilitating access and movement by the disabled occupant around the dwelling in order to enable him to care for a person who is normally resident in the dwelling and is in need of such care;

l) such other purposes as may be specified by order of the Secretary of State.

If people want to know what adaptations are available they can visit a Disabled Living Centre (DLC) where a whole range of equipment and adaptation items are on display. If they make an appointment a member of staff will help and let them try out different items. In Hampshire 'Design Options for a Versatile Environment' (DOVE) is an organisation of disabled people that goes even further and has model adapted rooms for people to view and try out. Telephone 01705 787788 for further information.

Adaptation: action that can be taken

1 Simple adaptations, such as a hand rail up the stairs, are often supplied with a minimum of fuss. Council housing departments or housing associations may fit them for their tenants on request. Social services departments may also organise their supply and fitting free of charge, in any tenure; or householders may choose, pay for, and have them fitted themselves.

2 For more complex adaptations, the normal process in all tenures is to ask social services to carry out an assessment for adaptations. This is usually carried out by occupational therapists because of their specialist training and they will work with the applicant to develop options and to agree a solution which meets their needs and wishes.

After assessment, funding has to be identified. This is a complex area, and one where dialogue and sharing of costs between social services authorities and housing agencies is necessary. Details on the funding of adaptations are to be found in Heywood and Smart (1996).

Grants for adaptation

1 **The mandatory disabled facilities grant** (see table on home adaptation): this is now the only mandatory housing grant. Important changes from the provisions of the 1989 Local Government and Housing Act are:

• only the incomes of the applicant and partner, and parents if the disabled person is a child, will be subject to the test of resources – not the income of the owner of the property if that is someone different;

• grant is now mandatory for items relating to safety (Section 23(1)b); this may be important for service users with learning or behavioural difficulties, and for those with sensory impairment, as well as for older people requiring security measures or alteration to reduce hazards;

• the provision relating to lavatory and bathroom have been made absolutely clear – that the disabled person is entitled to access to and use of a lavatory and use of bath and/or shower in addition to use of a wash handbasin;

• there is no longer a requirement that a property receiving disabled facilities grant must also be made fit (ie, put into good repair throughout);

Cooperation between housing and social services on disabled facilities grant funding

The social services top-up budget can be crucial in obtaining grant funding [including 60% government subsidy] that might otherwise be lost when an applicant cannot afford their share of the cost.

Also £20,000 [the maximum grant] is sometimes not enough to pay for adaptations needed especially if there is more than one disabled member of the household or where there are major difficulties with the house because of limited space, style of construction etc.

In some authorities, social services pay the first few thousand (the amounts vary) of all applicants' contributions to disabled facilities grant, and consider further help according to the merits of the case. Other social services departments have delegated to officers the power to top-up to an additional £20,000, and have allocated appropriate budgets.

Realistic budgets, delegated powers and agreements about how the costs of work over £20,000 are to be shared all help reduce delays for the person in urgent need of adaptations.

- part of each housing authority's budget allocation for private sector housing in England will be ring-fenced for disabled facilities grants; all mandatory and discretionary disabled facilities grants will have to come out of this Specified Capital Grant; the other part of the budget will be for all other grants, including Home Repair Assistance.

2 **Discretionary disabled facilities grant:** this may be used for the 'accommodation, welfare or employment' of the disabled applicant. The major change of the 1996 Act is that discretionary disabled facilities grant may now also be used to fund mandatory items if mandatory grant is insufficient. It will now become necessary for housing and social services authorities to agree which of them should give the funding in such circumstances as both have the powers, social services has the duty and shortage of resources may be a problem for both authorities.

Maximising use of the existing adapted housing stock

Adaptation is an issue for those who rent just as much for those who own. Landlords, including local authorities and housing associations, sometimes express concern not only at the cost of home adaptation but also at the likelihood that the next tenant will have no need for the adaptation work. All housing agencies should classify and identify adapted property in their housing stock/needs registers. A number of schemes now exist which attempt to make maximum use of adapted properties which become available by matching them to households seeking to move to an already adapted property. Examples of such schemes are the Kent Disabled Persons Accommodation Agency and the Sheffield Disability Housing Service.

---

3 **Home Repair Assistance:** up to a maximum of £2,000 for one grant and up to £4,000 in three years, is a suitable way of providing minor

adaptations. Circular 17/90 Annex 1 para 66 recommends that "steering disabled people to home repair assistance in appropriate cases will ensure they receive more speedy help than through the more complex procedures for DFG".

Test of resources for disabled facilities grant

This means test is prescribed by central government, and local housing authorities do not have the power to vary it. It is based on the principal of establishing how much an applicant should be able to afford themselves, and only giving grant for any sum more than this. Those on the lowest incomes will be assessed as being able to afford nothing, and will get 100% grant, but others may get no help. No account is taken of mortgage or other debt commitments, so the applicants are often quite unable to pay their contribution because the money that is supposed to pay for the loan is already being used to pay the mortgage. This is why social services will often find cases of hardship among disabled facilities grant applicants, especially those with mortgages.

Some social services departments ask disabled facilities grant applicants to apply to a bank or building society for the loan of their assessed contribution, and to bring the letter of refusal so that the need for top-up can be demonstrated.

People should be encouraged to apply for disabled facilities grant even if they have to pay for all or most of the work themselves. This is because if they need more work at a later date, provided the subsequent work is within the 'notional loan' period (5 or 10 years), the money they have paid out first time will be deducted from any subsequent contribution – but *only* if they complete the disabled facilities grant procedure first time around.

A. Name of grant	B. Purposes	C. Who eligible	D. Terms	E. Conditions
Mandatory disabled facilities grant	To facilitate use by disabled people of their homes Specifically to provide • access to building • making dwelling safe for disabled persons or others • access to and provision of living room, bedroom, lavatory, bathroom (including use of bath and/or shower) and wash handbasin • providing suitable cooking facilities and suitable power, lighting and heating controls • improving or providing suitable heating system • movement around dwelling in order to care for someone • other purposes as may be specified by the Secretary of State	Anyone over 18 in any tenure who is either disabled themselves or needs the grant to allow them to adapt the house for a disabled person. The definition of disabled person for purposes of this grant is given at Section 100 of the 1996 Housing Grants, Construction and Regeneration Act. It includes a very broad range of older and disabled people, including disabled children	Mandatory for the purposes defined in Section 23, a-l of the 1996 Housing Grants, Construction and Regeneration Act. Maximum grant £20,000 (but NB discretionary grant for mandatory purposes may be added on). Test of resources as prescribed by the Secretary of State. Housing authorities must be satisfied that works are: (a) 'necessary and appropriate' and (b) 'reasonable and practicable'. In deciding '(a)' they shall consult the social services authority if it is a different authority. Payment of grant may in exceptional cases (ie, where it would not cause hardship to the applicant) be deferred for 12 months from the date of application	Disabled person (or parent if the disabled person is a child) must complete a test of resources which takes into account their income and that of their partner or spouse. This means test does not take existing outgoings into account, and there are therefore serious problems for people with mortgages or other debts. DoE Circular (4)97 provides for test of resources to be applied to people over 16 and under 19, in receipt of Income Support and no longer at school, in their own right, even if they are living with their parents
Discretionary disabled facilities grant	Either to augment a mandatory grant for purposes described above or to make the building suitable for the 'accommodation, welfare or employment' of the disabled occupant	As above	Discretionary Test of resources as above	

Note: This table is provided only as a guide. Full details need to be checked in the 1996 Housing, Grants, Construction and Regeneration Act, Part I and in subsequent Circulars.

Interpreting disabled facilities grant legislation

For professionals from all disciplines the guidance provided in Department of the Environment Circular 17/96 in Chapter 7 and Annex 1 is likely to be most helpful. The Circular is a very positive document stressing the enabling and flexible nature of the grants legislation. The sections on disabled facilities grant constantly emphasise the importance of involving the disabled person:

... the needs of the disabled occupant are paramount within the framework of what can be offered. (see Circular 127/96, ch 7, para 6.1)

The central purpose of disabled facilities grant is stated clearly in Annex 1, para 16:

In considering applications for grant towards such work (ie, works eligible for mandatory disabled facilities grant) the presumption should be that the occupant should have reasonable access into his home, to the main habitable rooms within the home – namely the living room and bedroom and to a bathroom or shower room in which there are suitable facilities for washing and/or showering.

Paragraph 49 of the same Annex stresses the overall objective of disabled facilities grants – "to give disabled people a degree of independence in the home".

Adaptation works would not have achieved their objective within a care package if the disabled person does not gain an acceptable degree of independence, where possible, or where the disabled person remains dependent upon the care of others, where the adaptation does not significantly ease the burden of the care.

Other paragraphs give helpful examples of how the provisions may be used to help those with sensory impairment or behavioural problems (paras 27, 17, 18 and 19) and help commend the use of expert advice for particular problems. There is also, throughout, a stress on the need for dialogue between housing and social services authorities and a problem solving approach to all the aspects of adaptation where responsibility is shared.

Examples of cooperation in planning, funding and implementing repairs and adaptations

Joint working is essential on a range of issues:

• jointly agreeing policies and procedures which set a clear framework for operational staff;

• making information available to those who need the service;

• assessment and specification;

• delivering a well coordinated, swift and user-friendly service from first enquiry to final inspection;

• ensuring that the building work is backed up by support services;

• using existing resources collaboratively to solve the problems of individuals.

Making more information available

Health and energy adviser
An energy adviser employed in the architects department of Newark and Sherwood District Council in Nottinghamshire has sought the help of health visitors in distributing energy conservation information to the people they visit. This can lead to a home visit by the energy adviser where she talks through measures which will help households stay warm at a reasonable cost.

Health, housing and social services
A project in Cardiff originally funded with health money from the King's Fund has made a video advertising services, including adaptations, for families from minority ethnic groups, and is working with housing and social services to help spread understanding from the authorities to the families and back again.

Assessment and specification

This is the core issue of joint working on adaptations and in most areas it works very well. Occupational therapists and environmental health officers either do joint visits, or have other established ways of accepting and trusting each other's professional skills. There are moves, too, to listen more carefully to what the service users want, and to have sufficient occupational therapy staff to be able to stress quality of assessments, not just the volume.

Good practice examples

In pilot projects in Essex, the social services department have been encouraging assessment staff to take longer and to improve the quality of assessment. This better identification of users' needs, with action on preventative measures, appears to be reducing the level of capital expenditure on adaptations.

In Epsom, Surrey, the social services department pays the cost of independent occupational therapists being employed within the Care and Repair agency. This arrangement helps to reduce demand and therefore waiting lists, and enables the agency to give an integrated service.

In Wakefield, a unitary authority, the housing department, has not merged with social services but has taken over its powers in relation to assessment. It has also taken on those of environmental services in relation to grants in order to create a powerful adaptations and disability unit within the health and elderly services section of the housing department, dealing with all tenures. It has a budget of £2m and the principal occupational therapist employed by the housing department has the right to allocate a house and over-rule the area housing management.

The creation of a Derwentside Care and Repair agency reduced the occupational therapist waiting list by about 40%. This seems to be a fairly widespread experience. If occupational therapists are filling in grant application forms, drawing up schedules of work and helping to supervise builders, they are not free to get on with the work where their skills and training are essential. Setting up an agency is a good way of ensuring that scarce occupational therapy skills are used most efficiently.

Delivering a well coordinated, swift and user friendly service

The Pieda report (1996) on the disabled facilities grant system outlined mechanisms for improving liaison at the operational level:

- the creation of joint teams;

- regular liaison meetings between social services staff and grants staff; this probably needs to occur both at a senior level to discuss policy, and at a lower level to discuss particular cases;

- many authorities have found it useful to undertake joint training so that both social services authority staff and housing authority staff understand the responsibilities of staff in the other authority and the way in which that authority operates;

- joint visits where the adaptations to be provided are likely to be complex and require a technical input; the contact that such visits afford also help to build up personal relationships between staff;

- common information systems; authorities could examine establishing common information systems (databases) that would allow staff in one authority, for example, to identify what stages in the enquiry process the client has reached.

Examples of cooperation

Design options for a versatile environment (DOVE)
Background
DOVE originated from discussions within the Housing and Independent Living group of Portsmouth Disability Forum. Members of the group, consisting of disabled people and representatives from statutory and voluntary agencies, heard from disabled people about the lack of users involvement in the design and specification of adaptations to their homes, often resulting in dissatisfaction in the completed work. This problem, and the difficulty of identifying suitable accommodation for disabled people wishing to move house for any reason, were highlighted in a conference in Portsmouth in 1994. Following the conference a steering group was formed to manage the setting up of a Resource Centre. DOVE opened to the public in December 1995, with an official opening in July 1996.

Location
Based in Cosham, Portsmouth, DOVE is available to residents of Hampshire and adjacent counties.

Structure
DOVE became incorporated as a company limited by guarantee in 1996. The directors and management group are all disabled people and there is also an advisory group of professionals from statutory agencies. The staff comprises a manager, who is an occupational therapist, an office administrator and a housing coordinator.

Functions
DOVE offers advice and information on all aspects of housing options for disabled people. Individuals visiting or contacting the centre can see and try out products to help them make informed choices about their present and future needs. The occupational therapist works with disabled people and professionals in the design, planning and implementation of adaptations. The housing coordinator develops links with housing providers to match available properties to those people with housing needs, and provides practical advice and support to individuals moving into the community.

Users
The service is provided, free of charge, to all disabled people in Hampshire. A range of professionals involved in housing design and adaptation also use the services.

Funding
DOVE has been funded by Hampshire Social Services and Portsmouth City Council and is seeking service agreement with both authorities for continued funding for the service. The occupational therapy post is a permanent secondment from social services and the building is provided by social services. The office administrator and housing coordinator post are funded for one year by Portsmouth City Council.

Contact: DOVE, c/o PCMI, Northern Road, Cosham, Portsmouth, PO6 3EP, Telephone 01705 787788

In Cheltenham, a 'practitioners' liaison group' meets every six weeks to coordinate the process of adaptation. Members include grant officers, surveyors, local authority housing managers, occupational therapists and in difficult cases, perhaps the local authority repairs inspector or other technical officers. The meeting is chaired by the Cheltenham Care and Repair manager. The agenda is arranged so that core business is discussed in the middle and the occupational therapists from east and west Cheltenham respectively attend either the first hour plus the core, or the core plus the second hour, so as to use their time most effectively. The meeting has a case list with key dates:

First referral
Inspection/assessment
Grant approval
Work ongoing

so that delays can be identified and action allocated as appropriate.

The Care and Repair manager says that the group acts as an ongoing training exercise for all parties involved in adaptations as the process is so complex and communication so important.
[Further information – Cheltenham Care and Repair, Telephone 01242 512280.]

Liaison group policy issues sometimes arise. A policy coordination group of the more senior practitioners now also meets to refer these questions up to a higher level.

Backing up repairs and adaptation with support services

Effective adaptations have the capacity to reduce the demands on carers or to make their caring tasks easier. They can also reduce the need for support services. For example, if a coal fire is replaced with a gas or electric fire, there is no need for a daily fire-lighting service. However, it is important that adaptations continue to be seen as only one important element of a good community care package which may also include domestic support and help with essential home maintenance.

Good practice examples

> In Gillingham, Special Transitional Grant has been used to establish a handy person scheme providing a speedy response, at minimal cost, to the problems experienced by older people needing small repairs to their homes. (Source: Bradford, Mares and Wilkins, 1994)

> Sheffield Stay Put (a Home Improvement Agency) was approached by the Health Authority's health promotion centre to operate jointly a home safety check scheme. Funding has been obtained from Joint Finance to employ a half-time project manager, two field workers and clerical assistance.
>
> The scheme will offer a comprehensive home safety check to people aged over 60, whatever their housing tenure. It will involve room by room examination which will identify possible hazards, eg, lack of stair rail, poor lighting and unguarded fires. It will also:
>
> * refer unsafe hearing appliances to the gas and electricity companies;
> * check connection on old electrical appliances and secure loose cables;
> * install smoke detectors;
> * fasten down loose floor coverings;
> * install security locks on doors and windows.
>
> The scheme will refer on for adaptations and equipment, in cases of identified need.
>
> Source: Bradford, Mares and Wilkins (1994)

> **Meeting the needs of people with complex multiple disabilities in Manchester: community learning disability teams**
> **Four community learning disability teams** made up of social workers/care managers, learning disability nurses, psychologists, speech therapists, occupational therapists, physiotherapists, domiciliary care organisers and staff, and administrative and clerical staff. These staff (about 25 in each team) assess the needs of individuals and their families and plan, organise, and deliver the support they require. There are also staff who provide additional support for people whose behaviour presents challenges.
>
> The benefits of the community learning disability team fieldworkers' approach are illustrated by work with three young men – one Sikh, one Muslim, one white British – with major physical and learning disabilities who live in an ordinary bungalow. Specialised support and intensive therapy are provided by direct care staff under the supervision of a speech and language therapist and a physiotherapist. Special equipment (eg, exercise mat, hoists, oxygen and medical aids) is provided in the house in a way that avoids producing a medical environment. The decoration of the house reflects the different cultural backgrounds and individual personalities of the three tenants. This approach ensures maximum achievement through constant input and continuous skilling and monitoring of staff.

Conclusion

In the last few years, there have been many hard-working groups of people in different parts of the country who have striven to make links between housing, health and social services in the provision of better repaired and well-adapted housing. Joint working, joint training, secondment of staff, use of HIAs, joint departments and the use of Joint Finance, as well as better planning, have all contributed to a growing sense of a common purpose and some areas have become centres of excellence. The increasing involvement of Health Authorities is much to be welcomed.

Guide to further reading

Bradford, I., Mares, P. and Wilkins, N. (1994) *Home for good: making homes fit for community care*, Nottingham: Care and Repair. [A user-friendly mine of practical information on housing issues for health and social services personnel. Three separate sections are aimed at policy makers, practitioners and trainers respectively. Don't be put off by the heavy ring binder – take the sections out and use them separately.]

Care and Repair and College of Occupational Therapists (1994) *Pulling together: developing effective partnerships*, Nottingham: Care and Repair. [A joint statement on good practice.]

Carter, S. (1997) *Against the odds: London councils delivering housing services to disabled people*, London: London Housing Unit. [Very strong on planning and strategic thinking and on practical suggestions.]

Cowen, A. (undated 1996) *Taking care*, York: Joseph Rowntree Foundation for the Family Fund. [Publication offers general information about disabled children. Written for parents but useful to all sorts of practitioners. *Free to parents.*]

Department of the Environment (1996) *Private sector renewal: a strategic approach*, London: HMSO, Circular 17/96. [Provides detailed outline of the policy and practice implications of recent changes in the law governing improvement and adaptation grants.]

Heywood, F. (1994) *Adaptations: finding ways to say yes*, Bristol: SAUS Publications. [A practical guide to helping people through the maze of getting adaptations done.]

Heywood, F. (1996) *Managing adaptations*, Bristol: The Policy Press. [Available free from the ADSS Disability Committee, Telephone 0181 5476001. A guide designed to help social services achieve a positive approach to adaptation services in partnership with other key parties.]

Heywood, F. with Smart, G. (1996) *Funding adaptations: the need to cooperate*, Bristol: The Policy Press. [This gives a detailed profile of the current financial situation nationally and in 53 local authorities by unravelling the confusion of funding sources and legal responsibilities.]

Leather, P., Mackintosh, S. and Rolfe, S. (1994) *Papering over the cracks*, London: National Housing Forum. [Draws upon the English House Condition Survey and other sources to profile the extent of housing disrepair.]

Lewis, B. (1992) *Access for life*, Clay Cross: Derbyshire Coalition of Disabled People. [Presents the case for adaptable accessible homes in a barrier free environment.]

Meghani-Wise, Z. (1996) 'Why this interest in minority ethnic groups?', *Bristol Journal of Occupational Therapy*, October, vol 59, no 10. [A really useful introduction to cultural and religious issues affecting adaptation needs, including bibliography.]

National Children's Home (nd) 'Care for children with disabilities – a lifeline for the whole family' and 'Checklist of benefits and services for families caring for a child with disabilities at home'. [Free leaflets, Telephone 0171 226 2033. Also Publications Catalogue with several relevant publications.]

Pieda plc (1996) *An evaluation of the disabled facilities grants system*, London: HMSO. [A major study funded by the Department of the Environment, Transport and the Regions on the operation of the disabled facilities grant system.]

Social Services Inspectorate (1994) *Occupational therapy: the community contribution*, London: HMSO. [Telephone 01973 840250, Department of Health Distribution Centre. An important discussion of the pivotal role of occupational therapists in community care.]

Housing agencies and primary healthcare teams

module five

Objectives

1 To establish the circumstances in which primary healthcare and housing staff are required to work cooperatively in relation to individual cases.

2 To develop housing staff's understanding of the culture, functioning and environment of primary healthcare teams.

3 To develop primary healthcare teams' understanding of the culture, functioning and environment of housing agencies.

4 To identify the difficulties users, primary healthcare staff and housing staff experience with the interface between health and housing.

5 To highlight innovative ways in which these difficulties have been addressed at the operational level.

What is the primary healthcare team?

Although the detailed membership of primary healthcare teams vary, they are likely to look something like this example below:

Why work together?

• Housing can significantly affect the health and well-being of individuals.

• Changes in the health and fitness of an individual may require changes in their housing arrangements to maximise the potential for independence and quality of life.

• The interplay between housing conditions and health status has particularly dire consequences for some groups of people, such as homeless people.

Homeless people age much faster than housed people, have much lower life expectancy and suffer disproportionately high levels of chest complaints, muscular skeletal problems, accidental injury and the health problems associated with poverty, cold and poor diet. (Llewellin and Murdock, 1996)

The complex interaction between housing conditions and the physical environment, social circumstances and health status which leads to the deterioration in the health and well-being of individuals does not easily translate into the responsibility of an identifiable professional or agency. As a result there is a need for housing, social services and primary healthcare staff to work together to ensure that their particular knowledge and

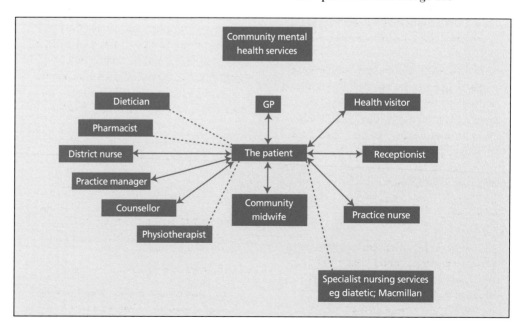

expertise are used to solve the problems of individuals and households with interconnected health, welfare and housing needs.

- Service users and carers in contact with one agency should be able to rely on that agency having knowledge of, information on and good working practices with all other key agencies relevant to addressing health, care and support and housing needs. Individuals should not be left to make the connections themselves.

- Such joint working should be open, offer choice and be 'user friendly'.

When to work together

There are a number of circumstances affecting individuals or households when primary healthcare workers and housing staff may need to work together. The main occasions are as follows:

During the process of housing allocation: this may apply either

- to individuals or households seeking to move into 'social' housing from the privately rented market or from owner-occupation or from a state of homelessness; or

- to those who are already occupying 'social' housing and are seeking to be rehoused within this housing tenure.

In both these circumstances the prompt which triggers some form of joint working is when a medical or health condition or a functional problem is seen by some key party as contributing to the need for the individual or household to be housed or rehoused. Such individuals are part of the routine workload of many housing staff but are not a core part of the workload of most primary healthcare teams.

In practice, this relationship between primary healthcare and housing staff is often mediated through a third party, a medical assessor or advisor to the housing agency. Increasingly requests

from housing staff for medical information from GPs is organised through such medical advisers. (A detailed account of the workings of medical advisors in housing agencies is provided by Smith et al, 1993 – see Guide to further reading.)

Enabling individuals or households to 'stay put' in their own homes: this can apply to individuals in all forms of housing tenure who require adaptations or repairs to be carried out to their existing housing. The joint working may be prompted by a change in the health status of an individual or a deterioration in the property which becomes a hazard to the health or safety of the individual.

Since the major group who tend to experience increasing health-related problems over time are older people and since they also tend to own housing in a poor state of repair, primary healthcare teams are likely as a matter of routine to come into contact with older people who need help to 'stay put'. Housing staff, in order to address such needs, frequently require the support of social services and occupational therapists.

The assessment of individuals for care and support packages who have health and housing needs: this involves situations of care management assessment where the assessment expertise of health and housing need to be drawn in. However, only a minority of the people known to housing and primary healthcare teams will be known to social services (eg, 97% of the population is registered with a GP).

Requesting joint working

The prompt for cooperation between primary healthcare teams and housing staff may therefore be triggered by a range of individuals, which include:

- the person with the housing need;

- an informal carer who has a housing need relating to their caring role;

- a member of the primary healthcare team or health project worker;

- a member of a housing agency or housing project;

- social services staff.

It is therefore important that all aspects of the system for giving and receiving information are open and appropriate to the needs of this range of individuals.

What primary healthcare staff need to understand about housing

The policy context

Reproduced below is the section from **Module One** about the housing policy context to joint working, while the section on housing and mapping your locality from **Module Two** is also highly relevant.

Housing

1 Many people want to own their own homes and owner-occupation is now the dominant tenure. Alongside this the government is committed to supporting efficiently run social and private rented sectors.

2 The work of housing authorities (metropolitan authorities, district councils and London boroughs) has broadened and diversified in recent years:

i)   they have developed their enabling and strategic role;
ii) some local authorities have delegated their housing management services to an external organisation such as a private sector contractor, a managing agent or a tenant management organisation;
iii) some local authorities have transferred some or all of their housing stock usually to registered social landlords which include

housing associations (transfer has often been in the form of large-scale voluntary transfer or LSVT; by early 1997, there were over 50 LSVTs managing around 250,000 socially rented homes).

3 Social housing now:

i)   houses a high proportion of 'vulnerable' households;
ii) is allocated more on the basis of need.

4 The work of registered social landlords, such as housing associations, has involved:

i)   developing most new socially rented housing;
ii) a funding regime based upon a public–private partnership;
iii) an expanded role as providers of care and support services, including services purchased by health and social services.

5 There has been some revival in private renting – it remains a minority tenure but one that may be used by numerous people with community care needs.

6 'Special needs' housing schemes continue to make an important contribution to those with housing and support needs but they have come under increased criticism for their separation from mainstream provision.

7 Health and social services professionals often have a very narrow view of housing work. The Chartered Institute of Housing defines the following housing management tasks as being core competencies:

i)   Lettings, allocations, transfer and nominations
ii) Homelessness and housing advice
iii) Rent collection
iv) Rent arrears management
v)   Housing benefits work
vi) Tenant participation and consultation

vii) Repairs reporting, inspection and maintenance systems

viii) Voids management (ie, the management of empty property)

ix) Estate management

8 However, this is the only partial picture of the diversity of work that may be carried out by staff employed by housing providers. Social services and health staff will often need to have contact with care and support staff and with sheltered housing staff, whose work is not reflected in the above list and whose work may be funded from a variety of sources including contracts with social services and health purchasers. Important, yet frequently missing, players in housing/ homelessness and community care debates are environmental health officers, because of their pivotal roles in the home improvement grant system, home adaptations and in monitoring housing standards, including in the private rented sector. Care and Repair and/or Home Improvement Agency staff can also have an important role in advising elderly people and disabled people on improvement and adaptation issues. It also needs to be remembered that housing workers and other staff might be working for the local authority, a registered social landlord (the size and scope of which vary enormously) or a voluntary organisation.

Additional information

The primary function of housing agencies is to manage a particular 'stock' of housing and to allocate this to those individuals or households who request access to or a move within accommodation provided by that agency. Systems of awarding points and waiting lists have developed to allocate housing to those in greatest need since in many areas demand exceeds supply.

Housing agencies can only match needs of individuals and households to the existing stock of housing and lack flexibility to fine tune accommodation to specific needs. A priority – and, indeed, a performance indicator – for housing departments is the number of properties which are vacant and the length of time of these 'voids'. There is therefore a need to match people to existing vacant accommodation and, while sometimes in theory the agencies might hold housing which could address the needs of particular individuals, in practice this will only work out, at best, over fairly long timescales. This is very different from the culture and functioning of medical services where there is often more flexibility to deliver individualised care very quickly.

The points system for allocating housing is a 'blunt' instrument when applied to health-related issues. This has led, in part, to physical health and mobility problems being given more consideration than mental health problems. Allocation systems may include age criteria (where these apply they will vary between housing authorities), but regardless of age housing authorities must, by law, give reasonable preference in their schemes to households who meet the criteria for allocating housing. The criteria include medical or welfare needs for which additional preference should be allowed in allocation schemes. Although authorities must allocate housing according to their published scheme there is room for discretion in special cases.

The roles of housing staff and the training they receive are not geared generally to the provision of individual health and social care. However, the significant shift in the characteristics of individuals and households now in social housing means that housing staff are often likely to be the front-line contact for people with severe health problems, who may also be exhibiting signs of mental distress.

Housing agencies are not homogeneous entities and the various functions they undertake (repairs and maintenance, rent collection, allocations, homelessness, etc) are often the responsibility of different sections within the agency (see **Module Two**). This may also mean that not all departments and staff have access to a shared data base, so that information on individual cases, for example, may not be available to all workers. This raises issues relating to confidentiality.

Trigger questions for primary healthcare teams

- Do you know the main housing agencies offices in your area (local housing office; homelessness unit; housing associations; voluntary run hostels; housing advice service; contact point for grants, etc)?

- Do you have a contact name and number for each of these?

- Do you have simple accessible information about each?

- Do you know the eligibility criteria of relevant housing agencies?

- Do you know how applications are made to these agencies?

- Do you know how each agency requires information on the health/medical conditions of applicants?

- Do you know how priority is given to different medical conditions?

- Do you know whether agencies employ or use the services of some form of medical advisor?

- Have you in the past year sent a representative from your team to have a face-to-face meeting with staff in the housing agencies in your area?

- Do you know the roles of housing staff? (eg, is there a shared understanding between agencies as to the role of housing wardens?)

- Is there an explicit policy about confidentiality in relation to the sharing of information between and within agencies for which client consent is sought on every occasion?

- Is there a routine feedback mechanism to monitor how individual cases have progressed and how the working relations between agencies are functioning?

- Is there an agency in your area which is able to help older or vulnerable homeowners carry out repairs or adaptations to their homes (Care and Repair or Staying Put schemes)?

- Do you have links with the agencies dealing with homeless people (including voluntary run drop-in centres and local day centres), so that they have access to mainstream primary healthcare?

- Are you able to give patients the name and number of welfare rights workers, and lawyers who have a special interest in housing issues?

What housing staff need to know about GPs and primary healthcare teams

Module One provided a general introduction to the policy context within which NHS professionals work, while the section on healthcare agencies and mapping your locality in **Module Two** is also highly relevant. Below is a more specific look at GPs and primary healthcare teams.

1   GPs work as individuals with independent contractor status. Although a number of GPs may work together in a practice a GP is not accountable to another for their clinical work. GPs may refer their patients on to other professionals in the primary healthcare team, or refer on to secondary care. GPs may claim reimbursement of certain practice expenses and a range of fees and allowances from Health Authorities as prescribed in the Statement of Fees and Allowances.

2   The reforms which have taken place within the NHS since 1990 have dramatically affected the functioning of GPs and primary healthcare teams. In 1990 a new General Practitioner Contract was introduced and this placed a greater emphasis on GPs being involved in health promotion and preventive care. Specific targets were set, for example, for immunisations, and health checks were introduced for all people over 75 years.

3   The 1990 NHS and Community Care Act offered the possibility for GPs to become fundholders. This scheme has been extended to include smaller practices and more services so that by 1997/98 it is estimated that 57% of the population will be covered by fundholding practices controlling 11% of local healthcare funds. Housing staff can identify fundholding practices through the local Health Authority.

4   GPs' training is based predominantly on a medical model of health and places an emphasis on the diagnosis, treatment and prevention of ill-health for individual patients.

5   The list of patients for any practice, while restricted by access times and distances, does not relate to other administrative boundaries, and practices often draw patients from shared 'catchment' areas. Within this framework the housing circumstances of patients is not normally given a high priority in the issues which should and can be realistically addressed.

6   Over 97% of the population is registered with a GP although the percentage of homeless people registered is much smaller. All citizens have the right to be registered with a GP and this is the route to all forms of medical care, including inpatient and outpatient hospital treatment.

7   Patients are free to approach any GP and ask to be included in that doctor's list of patients. GPs can, however, decline to accept a person as a patient. This is usually because the doctor considers his list to be full or because the patient does not live within the desired practice area. GPs can also ask for patients to be removed from their list and are not legally obliged to provide an explanation. However, there is strong professional guidance about when such action is, and is not, appropriate. Homeless people have exactly the same rights of access to a GP as those with a permanent address and GPs are encouraged to accept them onto their lists. Doctors can choose to treat people who are not registered with them as temporary residents. If any person cannot find a GP to treat them the local Health Authority are obliged to help them, if necessary by assigning them to a GP.

8   GPs, along with opticians, dentists and pharmacists, are contracted to the Health Authority for the provision of services to the patients on their list.

9   The structure and relationships within primary healthcare teams are complex and have changed significantly over the last five years. Practice nurses (and the growing number of practitioner nurses) are employed by the GP and work almost entirely on the practice premises. Community health workers (midwives, health visitors, district nurses, community psychiatric nurses), may be attached to a general practice but are employed by an NHS trust. In addition, physiotherapists, chiropodists and counsellors may be employed by the practice.

10 A recent addition to primary healthcare teams are practice business managers. Some of these business managers also act as fund managers for GPs who have chosen to

be fundholders, or in some cases, the practice employs both a fund manager and a business manager.

11 In order to develop any collaborative working relations with a primary healthcare team it is essential to have the backing of the GPs since they lead the primary healthcare team. This does not, however, automatically mean that the joint working actually involves GPs on a day-to-day basis; there are other members of the team who may, in fact, be more suitable to liaise with over individual cases.

12 The timescales and the extent to which it is possible to produce a response tailored to the particular needs of an individual through direct access to services are inevitably different for housing staff and health professionals. The latter are more accustomed to rapid responses to changing health needs and flexibility to match the treatment to specific medical conditions. Within primary healthcare, an 'urgent' referral requires a response the same day and all the population can access the NHS 24 hours a day every day of the year.

Trigger questions for housing staff

- Do you know the practices locally within your area and how to find out about others?

- Do you have information on the number of doctors and the range of other staff working from each practice?

- Do you know which practices have a practice manager and the name of the managers?

- Do you have a contact in your local Health Authority who has knowledge of the general practices in your area?

- Has your agency in the last year had a face-to-face meeting with a representative from the local primary healthcare teams?

- Is there an explicit policy about confidentiality in relation to the

sharing of information between and within agencies for which client consent is sought on every occasion?

- Does your agency have a medical adviser and are you clear how to make effective use of them?

- Is there a routine feedback mechanism to monitor how individuals have progressed and how working relations between agencies are functioning?

Factors enabling the involvement of GPs

This list is derived from research undertaken on the involvement of GPs in community care (Leedham and Wistow, 1993). The points raised are, however, applicable to joint working with housing agencies. As indicated, GPs are critically important both in terms of their professional role and the lead position they have within the primary healthcare team.

- Demonstrate the benefits of new arrangements in terms of better outcomes for GPs' patients and a more cost effective use of resources.

- Develop awareness, understanding, vision and commitment among GPs.

- Specify clearly and practically how GPs can link into local assessment arrangements which make most effective use of their time.

- Allay fears of increased workloads. Emphasise that new arrangements enable GPs to work in ways which are different rather than requiring substantial amounts of additional work.

- Establish known contact points for each GP (who prefer to work consistently with a person known to them), who can provide easy access/referral together with a quick response.

- Build on methods of working that GPs currently favour and use – keep paperwork and bureaucratic procedures to a minimum and use simple and clear documentation whenever possible.

- Give feedback on referrals – demonstrate progress to encourage GPs to continue to develop their contribution.

Involving social services

As we have suggested earlier in this Module a high proportion of the individuals requiring primary healthcare teams and housing staff to work together to help them address their needs do not require the involvement of social services. There are circumstances, however, when it is essential to involve social services and some of these situations are summarised below:

- when the housing and health professionals are not sure of the community care needs of their client and so wish **to access a community care assessment;**

- the health and housing professionals wish **to access specific services provided or funded by social services,** such as home care or a place in a residential or nursing home;

- the housing and health professionals **need the help of a care manger to sort out the client's existing care package, to address issues relating to the distressing behaviour of neighbours known to social services or to assess whether the client's housing situation is exacerbating their social care needs.**

The Department of Health (1994) produced a report *The role of the GP and primary health care team* in the series of publications on 'Implementing caring for people'. This report discusses in some detail the issues raised by primary care workers collaborating with social services in relation to community care. Recommendations relating to strategic and operational level are made in each section.

Working at the interface: problems and solutions

[See pp 88-92. A number of projects are listed in brackets in the checklist column. These are profiled in the final section of this Module as examples of how key problems and issues are being tackled by operational staff on the ground.]

1 From the perspective of the service user and carer

Users and carers should be able to receive support and services from all agencies which meet the highest standards in relation to equal opportunity practices. Operational staff are dependent on policies, training and materials which enable them to operate to these high standards. It is not their responsibility to generate these resources but front-line staff must be consistently utilising those which are available. In addition, the position operational staff occupy in the interface between the agency and the user means that these staff have a crucial role to play in feeding back into the organisation the impact of policy and practices on users.

Issue

Service users should be able to rely on any agency contacted to carry out an holistic assessment and to make connections with other agencies relevant in addressing identified needs.

Checklist

Housing staff
- How are housing applicants given the opportunity to indicate their health and mobility needs? (Hub Project)

Primary healthcare teams
- How are patients given the opportunity to link housing problems to their health and mobility problems? (Wells Park Project)
- Are visits to the homes of patients used as an opportunity to explore housing issues?

All agencies
- Have you thought about developing a single assessment form which can be used within your agency and with other agencies to which referrals are made? (Hub Project)
- What is the policy in relation to the exchange of personal information between your agency and others with which you work? (Hub Project)

All service users and carers require accessible information on the circumstances in which they may seek help and the sources of support.

All agencies
- How do you ensure that people with learning difficulties, people with limited vision and hearing impairments receive information from sources which have been designed to make it easily accessible to them?
- Do you ensure that people with difficulties in reading in any language are receiving information which has been made available to them in other forms?
- What is the availability of translated materials, translators and advocates within your agency?
- How do you feed back any difficulties you become aware of as you address people's needs for information?
- Do you regularly check that information from other agencies is kept stocked up in your offices and that this information is given, when needed, to people contacting your agency?

Housing agencies
- What information is available on key health bodies, eg, AIDS/HIV, drug and alcohol services, GPs and health visitors, and do you know how your agency refers to these bodies? (Hub Project)

Primary healthcare teams
- How do you keep information on and contact names for the key housing bodies in your area, including those which deal with homeless people? (Wells Park Project)

Service users vary enormously in their abilities to express their views in different settings and may experience barriers even in approaching agencies.

All agencies
- Are you aware of the availability of any independent advocates and interpreters?
- How do you ensure that appropriate assessments are carried out during visits to the service users?
- Are women given the option of having a female visit them at home or at least having a female accompany male staff?
- What safeguards and choices are given to people who may be experiencing racial or sexual abuse in terms of the people and places they are asked to contact?
- Do you avoid making assumptions about individuals' access to phones or their ability to respond to phone calls made in English? (Wells Park Project)
- What arrangements are in place to cover situations when communication by phone is not possible or there are limitations in the user's command of written English or other first language?

Service users and carers sometimes find it difficult to speak openly in each others presence about their needs.

All agencies
- How do you give service users and carers the option of being assessed separately?
- How do you try to avoid using family members or main carers as proxies or interpreters for the views of individuals who have difficulty in expressing themselves?
- Do you allow carers to make a choice about the level of care they wish to provide?
- How do you take care to avoid stereotypes informing your view on the functions an individual can undertake and the level of support you consequently offer?

Housing agencies
- In the process of allocating housing, how do you ensure sensitivity to the possibility that there may be more than one person in the household whose health and mobility needs should be taken into consideration?
- Do you routinely consider improving access to or for informal carers as a criterion for rehousing? (MRU)

Service users are not always clear about the processes by which their needs are given priority or how they can challenge processes if they feel that they have not been fair.

All agencies
- How do you ensure service users are informed about the formal rules and procedures which apply to your practices? (MRU)
- In cases where you have elements of discretion are users informed of your line of accountability?
- How do you inform users of the standards that they can expect from your agency and are these standards monitored? (MRU)
- How are service users given accessible information on the complaints procedures which are open to them and are these systems monitored? (MRU)

2 From the perspective of housing staff and primary healthcare teams

Issue

Lack of understanding within the primary healthcare team about housing agencies and the nature of the local housing stock.
Primary healthcare teams do not appreciate the limited degree of choice housing agencies frequently have to meet individuals' needs.

What needs to be done and by whom

Primary healthcare team
- Ensure that at least one member of the team, either from local knowledge or 'training' from housing staff, understands the internal structure and functioning of the housing agencies and the housing stock which they manage.
- Ensure that advice given to patients and recommendation made to housing agencies are realistic in the light of what type of housing is available in the locality.

Housing agencies
- Circulate clear simple leaflets to primary healthcare teams so they know which agencies to refer patients on to and have a contact point at the agency. (MRU)
- Use a member of staff as a link with general practices and set up face-to-face visits through practice mangers, if available. (MRU)
- Contact the Health Authority to find out if any locality work is being developed with general practices and who has information about the practices to which your agency relates. (MRU)
- Strategically, representation on joint planning or joint commissioning teams or projects addressing certain Health of the Nation targets can be effective in increasing shared understanding. (MRU)

Communication of medical/health information on individual patients from the primary healthcare team to housing agencies.

GPs feel that the time they spend supporting patients' cases for housing are a waste of time. They do not appear to have much effect.

Housing agencies find that much of the information provided by doctors is untimely, inappropriate or irrelevant to the housing allocation process.

Housing staff
- Provide a form which specifies the type of information required.
- Provide clear information on the priority grading system in relation to medical/health circumstances to all primary healthcare teams.
- Make effective use of medical advisors and only seek information from GPs in cases where this is really necessary and GPs are properly briefed.
- Hold regular meetings when health and housing staff meet together to discuss individual cases. (Wells Park Project)
- 'Train' primary healthcare team members so that they understand the priority system and they provide information which is useful and you trust. This does not necessarily have to be a GP but could be a nurse or health project worker.

After referrals between agencies individuals 'disappear' and there is no knowledge of the outcome.

Jointly
- Arrangements should be made to feed back to each other on the progress and outcome of referrals. (Wells Park Project)

Healthcare staff in particular feel mental health issues are not given sufficient acknowledgement in housing allocation systems.

Jointly
- Face-to-face meetings between health and housing staff to discuss difficulties associated with individual people. This develops trust and understanding. (Wells Park Project; Castlefields Practice)
- Primary healthcare teams to work with medical assessors and housing staff to develop allocation systems more responsive to health/medical conditions. (Wells Park Practice)

Homeless people do not have access to medical care or have their health needs strongly reflected in the housing allocated to them.

Housing
- A single access point and/or form which allows both the health and housing needs of homeless people to be recorded. (Hub Project)
- Staff within an agency who can help an individual to make contact with health services/projects and in particular GPs.
- Health details kept confidential to the particular staff who fill in the health assessment form: this not to be done at 'the front desk' but in privacy when health assessment requested by the individual. (Hub Project)

Primary healthcare team
- Close working relationships to be developed with agencies or units who deal with homeless people.
- Arrangements made so that homeless people can have appointments with GPs in the routine way. (Hub Project)
- Priority to be given to the nature of the housing needed by homeless people in relation to their health problems rather than just a roof over their heads.

Health Authority
- Develop a system for allocating homeless people a local address so that it is easier to access mainstream primary healthcare.

Healthcare workers and users find it difficult to know the full range of housing agencies in any area and do not want to have to replicate filling in forms which are seeking similar information.

Housing agencies
- Consider developing a single registration form which is available in all welfare agencies and provides information which is common to all housing agencies in the area, or alternatively making an effective use of the local authority as an initial point of contact.

Issues addressed in practice

The Hub Project

General information about the Hub

Further information is available from Project Coordinator, The Hub, Schooner House, 13-17 Cumberland Street, St Pauls, Bristol BS2 8NL.

The Hub is a multi-agency project providing a single point of access to a number of organisations able to help and advice people in housing crisis. It primarily offers support to people in housing need whom the local authority has no duty to rehouse, such as single people. The agencies which work at Hub are the Cyrenians, Shelter, Avon Health, social services, careers service, City Council housing services, Deposit Bond Scheme and the Benefits Agency.

The health link workers are employed by the local Health Authority but do not have any formal medical or nursing training. They do not carry a case load and in general see only each client once. Assessments are carried out by the front of house team (the Cyrenians) using a single registration form. This covers basic health/care issues and all clients are asked whether they wish to talk with a health link worker. The registration form can be passed to all staff working in the project but the specific form relating to health assessment is confidential to the health link workers and is not handed on to to other workers if referrals are made to other agencies.

Homeless people getting requests for housing supported on health grounds

ISSUE

PRACTICE

All homeless people have an opportunity to flag up their concerns relating to health during the initial registration process. .

The health link workers act as advocates for individuals. They have direct contact with the housing officers based with Hub and know the way in which health issues relate to the priorities for housing allocation.

This project has been particularly effective in getting individuals who are vulnerable into housing. This means that the problems relating to mental health are addressed as well as those relating to mobility problems.

Homeless people accessing GPs and other forms of healthcare

ISSUE

PRACTICE

Many clients are not registered with a GP and the health workers will contact surgeries, make appointments and, if necessary, accompany clients. Referrals are also made to drug and alcohol projects and to a local mental health homeless liaison team. The clinics run by the local medical homeless project are also used if appropriate and open at the required time.

Medical Resource Unit

General information
Further information is available from Medical Resource Unit (MRU), Southwark Housing Department, 17 Bournemouth Road, London SE15 4UJ.

The MRU is responsible for carrying out medical assessments for people applying to Southwark Council for housing. A medical form is filled in by those who have a medical condition that affects the type of housing needed or need to move to look after someone who is ill or disabled.

The assessments are carried out by a nurse and frequently involve home visits.

The Unit also employs a health and housing advisor who liaises between health workers and the housing department.

Improving the level of awareness between health and housing staff

ISSUE

PRACTICE

The assessments are carried out by a nurse who is employed by the housing department. She works closely with the housing staff and understands the housing allocation process. This informs the way in which she presents the information on medical/health issues and the degree of trust which exists between housing and health staff.

The nurse assessor is a full-time post and this enables her to be involved in planning and strategic policy issues. She works jointly with housing and other health staff in groups addressing Health of the Nation targets relating to accident prevention, and has had input into housing regeneration projects.

The health and housing advisor visits local general practices, normally arranging the visit through the practice manager. He talks with primary healthcare staff about their problems in relation to housing and the role of the housing department. He also provides a leaflet which answers some of the questions primary healthcare workers most commonly ask in relation to housing issues.

In the face-to-face visits he particularly concentrates on ensuring that the practice knows that generalised letters of support are not needed but that patients with housing needs relating to health problems should be sent to the local housing office. He also explains the sort of timescales to which the housing departments works and that applicants are not lost, but that it may take several months to address their needs. He gives an overview on the nature of the local housing stock and the limitations this imposes on the department's ability to respond to particular needs.

ISSUE

PRACTICE

Informing the users on standards and complaint procedures

In its leaflet the MRU provides information for users on what they can do if they disagree with the medical decision made. In addition, the Unit provides a service standards document which sets out the targets to which the service aims to work and the method of complaining if things go wrong.

Wells Park Health Project: housing forum

General information
Further information is available from Wells Park Health Project, Wells Park Road, Sydenham, London.

The Health Project is attached to a general practice and was established as a result of the enthusiasm of the principal GP who continues to have a strong commitment and involvement with it. The Project works with the local community addressing particular needs, and with individual patients who are referred to them by the general practice.

The housing forum meets about every six weeks and involves health project workers and staff from the local housing office. The health workers flag up in advance the individuals about whom they have some concerns in relation to their progress through the housing assessment process.

ISSUE

PRACTICE

Improving the responsiveness of the housing allocation process to the health needs of individuals

Individuals who are referred to the Project are given wide-ranging support. This includes counselling and guidance relating to debts and childcare, for example. Those who have a housing problem are supported by the Project workers with such matters as filling in forms, and presenting their 'case' in the most effective way. This may involve a great deal of support for some people where translations or special arrangements to accommodate hearing difficulties are needed, or where the individual is intimidated by or angry with the bureaucratic procedures.

The Project workers will raise concerns with the housing staff at the forum over individuals who have not the energy nor the skills to follow up applications themselves but where there is some urgency (eg, for post-operative cancer patients), or where the individual is vulnerable and this is not apparent in the forms. In particular, they have been trying to get more account taken of clients' stress and related illnesses which are not recognised by the points system. In such instances the Project workers are acting as advocates for the individuals, with their consent.

Improving working relations between housing and health workers

ISSUE

PRACTICE

An additional benefit from the face-to-face meetings between health workers and housing staff is that over time a much higher level of trust develops and they understand better the nature of the issues with which each agency is dealing. In particular, housing staff develop a greater understanding of the nature of health problems which are not purely physical in origin and that addressing such issues can make a significant difference to the quality of life for an individual or household.

Health staff gain a knowledge of the local housing stock and the range of options available to the housing staff. They also understand the points allocation system and can better support individuals in presenting information in a way that can be used more effectively by the housing staff.

Both groups of staff get more satisfaction and incentive to maintain the forum as a result of receiving feedback on the outcome of their joint working. The forum is also being used as a platform to work towards developing a better system for GPs providing information for medical/health assessments. This should lead to GPs' concerns about the present weakness of this system being heard directly and addressed by the medical advisors to the housing department.

Primary care for homeless people team
(Camden and Islington Health Authority)

General information
Further information is available from the Coordinator, Primary Care for Homeless People Team, Camden and Islington Health Authority, 3rd Floor, Jacob House, 3-5 Cynthia Street, London N1 9JF.

Primary care for homeless people is a well established multi-disciplinary team funded by Camden and Islington Health Authority, working to improve access to local health services by homeless people in Camden and Islington. The guiding principle for all the work of the primary care for homeless people team is that good quality healthcare is a right for all individuals. The team comprises a coordinator, administrative support, GP facilitator (locum), clinical nurse specialists, health and housing link worker, health development worker, UCL hospitals discharge link worker.

GPs offer sessions for homeless people in various local centres. A hairdresser also offers sessions for homeless people.

The primary care for homeless people team aims to:

- treat all individuals in a non-judgemental way;

- ensure the services are accessible to all homeless people, regardless of their race, colour, gender, sexuality, age, disability or religion;

- improve the health of homeless people in an holistic way;

- enable individuals to make informed choices about their health and help to empower them to take action.

ISSUE

PRACTICE

Improving access to primary healthcare for homeless people

The team works within a wide interpretation of homelessness encompassing people who ae sleeping out or living in any form of temporary accommodation. There are approximately 10,000 homeless people living in Camden and Islington, representing almost 3% of the area's population.

The team has two roles:

- to provide healthcare for homeless people who do not have a doctor;

- to improve access to health services by homeless people.

Outreach sessions: held in day centres, drop-ins, nightshelters and hostels used by single homeless people and homeless families to provide direct access to medical care and to health advice, information, advocacy and support.

Advocacy: where people are given advice, information, support and practical help with using local services, eg, registering with a GP, finding a dentist, going to an outpatient appointment.

Development work: by making links between agencies (hostels, hotels, day centres) which have contact with homeless people and their local health services.

Training: sessions on 'Health and homelessness' are provided for health workers and a range of other disciplines, and the team accepts placements of medical students, student nurses, health visitors, etc.

Joint working: through ongoing joint working with statutory authorities to bring to their attention gaps in services and lack of access and to suggest ways in which service delivery/provision could be improved so that more homeless people are able to use them.

Information

- through continued working with service providers to ensure that information about their services, and how to use them, reaches homeless people;

- by providing information for use by agencies – *Directory of services for homeless people in Camden and Islington; How to get a doctor* leaflet and an *Information pack for GPs* which details advice and support services.

Guide to further reading

Arblaster, L. and Hawtin, M. (1993) *Health and housing and social policy*, Socialist Health Association. [Describes the relationship between health and housing and recent policies on social housing.]

Department of Health (1994) *Implementing caring for people, the role of the GP and primary health care team*, London: Department of Health. [A review of the developing role of GPs and primary healthcare teams in the implementation of the community care reforms.]

Ham, C. (1994) *Management and competition in the new NHS*, Oxford: Redcliffe Medical Press. [Provides a clear guide to and assessment of the reforms within the NHS since 1990.]

Khan, S. (1997) *Today's concerns and bleak tomorrow's*, London: Service Access to Minority Ethnic Communities (SAMEC). [A national study of the housing and health needs of older people from West Indian, Pakistani, Bangladeshi and Indian Communities – further information available from the author at the School of Urban Development and Policy, South Bank University.]

Leedham, I. and Wistow, G. (1993) 'Just what the doctor ordered', *Community Care*, 7 January. [A summary of how welfare professionals can engage with GPs.]

Llewellin, S. and Murdock, A. (1996) *Saving the day*, CHAR (Housing Campaign for Single People, 5-15 Cromer Street, London WC1H 8LS). [Underlines the importance of primary healthcare to single homeless people.]

Smith, S. et al (1993) *Housing provision for people with health and mobility needs, guide to good practice*, Department of Geography, University of Edinburgh. [Offers a guide to good practice based upon their extensive research on the limitations and variations of present practice.]

Thompson, K. et al (1995) *Mental health care: a guide for housing workers*, London: Mental Health Foundation. [This is a clear manual for housing workers which developed out of a training programme. It gives information on different forms of mental illness and mental healthcare provision. It also provides advice on how to communicate with people in mental distress.]

Winn, L. (ed) (1990) *Power to the people – the key to responsive services in health and social care*, London: King's Fund Centre. [Provides illustrations of how to increase user involvement for carers, older people, black and minority ethnic groups, people with learning disabilities and people with mental health problems.]

Hospital admission and discharge

module six

Objectives

1 To assist the process of a safe and timely discharge from hospital for the well-being of the service user.

2 To identify the problems experienced by social workers or other hospital-based staff in securing the rapid provision of suitable housing or an adapted home environment for their clients who are to be discharged from hospital.

3 To identify the problems experienced by the housing department and other housing agency workers at the interface with health and social services personnel at the points of hospital admission and discharge.

4 To provide guidelines for effective communication across the above agencies in relation to hospital admission and discharge and supply helpful trigger questions, checklists and suggestions for overcoming difficulties in achieving satisfactory housing and home environment outcomes for patients being discharged from hospital.

The context of hospital admission and discharge

This workbook focuses upon the interface between health, social services and **housing agencies** relating to the **housing** dimensions of hospital admission and discharge and should be viewed in the context of the care management process set out in the 1990 NHS and Community Care Act. The housing dimension needs to be specifically included as an integral part of the care management process because:

• adequate housing is an essential contributor to good health;

• provision, adaptation and renovation of suitable housing are key components of a system of comprehensive care;

• it is at the crucial stage of *admission*, rather than just discharge, that hospital-based staff need an awareness of the housing dimensions of a patient's needs;

• an individual who has undergone a major life change with illness may find that it triggers a change in housing need;

• the housing circumstances of people with an ongoing, chronic illness need to be monitored as these may contribute significantly to constant readmission; in such circumstances, the alertness of hospital staff to such a need should trigger an early assessment and referral for a housing solution;

• with regard to older people, there is a risk of inappropriate discharge, particularly where the patient or family/friends may have unrealistic expectations about care delivery in the sheltered or extra care environment or where the additional care requirements may be outside the existing contract between the housing provider and social services.

From **service users'** point of view, the need for attention to the housing dimension of hospital admission and discharge is very clear because:

• there is a risk that their stay in hospital will be prolonged;

• there is a risk that they will have to be readmitted;

• there is a risk of drift into residential care;

• in the case of lone individuals, particularly those admitted to hospital suddenly, there is a risk of loss of the home if, for example, no one is paying the rent, an unprotected property gets vandalised or squatters move in.

Assessment and care management

Since 1993, social services have been the lead agency in coordinating assessments for care in the community. This includes the hospital discharge of individuals who have complex and continuing health and social care needs. In such cases, the care management process will often involve a multi-disciplinary assessment coordinated by a care manager or other social worker. Where a housing dimension has been identified, housing agencies need to be connected into the process either by ward staff, the care manager/social worker or by an occupational therapist – whichever is relevant.

It is the liaison function with the sphere of housing which is considered here – a relationship not generally spelled out in detail in most locally agreed policies on discharge.

This workbook assumes that health and social services personnel in hospitals are already implementing national requirements for a jointly agreed and comprehensive process of discharge planning and provision. If they are not, a summary of these requirements is given below, but fuller reference to Henwood's *Hospital discharge workbook* (Department of Health, 1994) is recommended.

[The *Hospital discharge workbook* is available, free of charge, from BAPS, The Health Publications Unit Storage and Distribution Centre, Heywood Stores, Manchester Road, Heywood, Lancaster OL10 2PZ.]

Policy requirements for hospital discharge

National policy on hospital discharge is set out in Circulars HC(89)5, HSG(95)8 and LAC(95)5. The policy guidance (LAC(96)7) on the 1995 Carers (Recognition and Service) Act 1995 also covers hospital discharge arrangements. The Patient's Charter standards on the discharge of patients from hospital state that:

Before you are discharged from hospital, you can **expect** a decision to be made about how to meet any needs you may continue to have. Your hospital will agree arrangements with agencies such as community nursing services and local authority social services departments. You and, if you agree, your carers, will be involved in making these decisions and will be kept up to date with information at all stages.

What hospital social services staff need to know about housing
The policy context

Reproduced below is the section from **Module One** about the housing policy context to joint working, while the section on housing and mapping your locality from **Module Two** is also highly relevant.

Housing

1 Many people want to own their own homes and owner-occupation is now the dominant tenure. Alongside this the government is committed to supporting efficiently run social and private rented sectors.

2 The work of housing authorities (metropolitan authorities, district councils and London boroughs) has broadened and diversified in recent years:

i)   they have developed their enabling and strategic role;
ii) some local authorities have delegated their housing management services to an external organisation such as a private sector contractor, a managing agent or a tenant management organisation;
iii) some local authorities have transferred some or all of their housing stock usually to registered social landlords which include

housing associations (transfer has often been in the form of large-scale voluntary transfer or LSVT; by early 1997, there were over 50 LSVTs managing around 250,000 socially rented homes).

3 Social housing now:

i)   houses a high proportion of 'vulnerable' households;
ii) is allocated more on the basis of need.

4 The work of registered social landlords, such as housing associations, has involved:

i)   developing most new socially rented housing;
ii) a funding regime based upon a public–private partnership;
iii) an expanded role as providers of care and support services, including services purchased by health and social services.

5 There has been some revival in private renting – it remains a minority tenure but one that may be used by numerous people with community care needs.

6 'Special needs' housing schemes continue to make an important contribution to those with housing and support needs but they have come under increased criticism for their separation from mainstream provision.

4 Health and social services professionals often have a very narrow view of housing work. The Chartered Institute of Housing defines the following housing management tasks as being core competencies:

i)   Lettings, allocations, transfer and nominations
ii) Homelessness and housing advice
iii) Rent collection
iv) Rent arrears management
v)   Housing benefits work
vi) Tenant participation and consultation

vii) Repairs reporting, inspection and maintenance systems
viii) Voids management (ie, the management of empty property)
ix)   Estate management

8 However, this is only a partial picture of the diversity of work that may be carried out by staff employed by housing providers. Social services and health staff will often need to have contact with care and support staff and with sheltered housing staff, whose work is not reflected in the above list and whose work may be funded from a variety of sources including contracts with social services and health purchasers. Important, yet frequently missing, players in housing/ homelessness and community care debates are environmental health officers, because of their pivotal roles in the home improvement grant system, home adaptations and in monitoring housing standards, including in the private rented sector. Care and Repair and/or Home Improvement Agency staff can also have an important role in advising elderly people and disabled people on improvement and adaptation issues. It also needs to be remembered that housing workers and other staff might be working for the local authority, a registered social landlord (the size and scope of which vary enormously) or a voluntary organisation.

Additional information (reproduced from Module Five)

The primary function of housing agencies is to manage a particular 'stock' of housing and to allocate this to those individuals or households who request access to or a move within accommodation provided by that agency. Systems of awarding points and waiting lists have developed to allocate housing to those in greatest need, since in many areas demand exceeds supply.

Housing agencies can only match needs of individuals and households to the existing stock of housing and lack flexibility to fine tune accommodation to specific needs. A priority – and, indeed, a performance indicator – for housing departments is the number of properties which are vacant and the length of time of these 'voids'. There is therefore a need to match people to existing vacant accommodation and, while sometimes in theory the agencies might hold housing which could address the needs of particular individuals, in practice this will only work out, at best, over fairly long time scales. This is very different from the culture and functioning of medical services where there is much greater flexibility to deliver individualised care very quickly.

The points system for allocating housing is a 'blunt' instrument when applied to health related issues. This has led, in part, to physical health and mobility problems being given more consideration than mental health problems. Allocation systems may include age criteria (where these apply they will vary between housing authorities), but regardless of age housing authorities must, by law, give reasonable preference in their schemes to households who meet the criteria for allocating housing. The criteria include medical or welfare needs for which additional preference should be allowed in allocations schemes. Although authorities must allocate housing according to their published scheme there is room for discretion in special cases.

The roles of housing staff and the training they receive are not geared generally to the provision of individual health and social care. However, the significant shift in the characteristics of individuals and households now in social housing means that housing staff are often likely to be the front-line contact for people with severe health problems, who may also be exhibiting signs of mental distress.

Housing agencies are not homogeneous entities and the various functions they undertake (repairs and maintenance, rent collection, allocations, homelessness, etc) are often the responsibility of different sections within the agency (see **Module Two**). This may also mean that not all departments and staff have access to a shared data base – so that information on individual cases, for example, may not be available to all workers. This raises issues relating to confidentiality.

Trigger questions for hospital ward and social services staff

• Do you know the main housing agencies offices in your area (local housing office; homelessness unit; housing associations; voluntary run hostels)?

• Do you have a contact name and number for each of these?

• Do you have simple written information about each?

• Do you know the eligibility criteria of relevant housing agencies?

• Do you know how applications are made to these agencies?

• Do you know how each agency requires information on the health/medical conditions of applicants to be considered?

• Do you know how priority is given to different medical conditions?

• Do you know whether agencies employ or use the services of some form of medical advisor?

• Have you in the past year sent a representative from your team to have a face-to-face meeting with staff in the housing agencies in your area?

• Do you know the roles of housing staff? (eg, is there a shared understanding between agencies as to the role of housing wardens/sheltered housing staff?)

- Is there an explicit policy about confidentiality in relation to the sharing of information between and within agencies for which client consent is sought on every occasion?

- Is there a routine feedback mechanism to monitor how individual cases have progressed and how the working relations between agencies are functioning?

- Is there an agency in your area which is able to help older or vulnerable homeowners carry out repairs or adaptations to their homes? (Care and Repair or Staying Put schemes?)

- Do you have links with the agencies dealing with homeless people so that you can coordinate the housing assistance they can offer with social services and community health services and hence discharge the patient safely?

- Are you able to give patients the name and number of welfare rights workers and lawyers who have a special interest in housing issues?

What housing staff need to know about hospitals and hospital discharge

Module One provided a general introduction to the policy within which NHS professionals work, while the section on healthcare agencies and mapping your locality in **Module Two** is also highly relevant. Below is a more specific look at hospitals and hospital discharge.

Your local hospitals are likely to be organised broadly into:

- acute district general hospitals (perhaps catering for certain specialities and geographical catchment areas);

- acute specialty hospitals (eg, spinal and head injuries or cancer; children or women);

- local and community hospitals (care of elderly people; maternity; respite care; rehabilitation);

- mental health hospitals;

- hospitals for people with learning disabilities.

NHS trusts are the bodies which run the hospitals and often a number of hospitals are clustered within one trust. The trusts are independent of the Health Authority and have their own management structure with a chairperson, hospital board and a chief executive.

Some NHS trusts combine the provision of hospital services with the delivery of community health services (nursing care, services and supplies to people in their own homes; day centres; day hospitals, etc) and mental health services. In other cases, community health services exist as a separate trust and, while mental health services may be included, sometimes these services are also delivered by a separate trust. Ambulance services may be a separate trust or part of another trust along with other services.

Within the hospital, the consultant takes the decisions about admission and discharge to inpatient beds. Ward nursing staff (individual inpatients have a 'named nurse' with responsibility for their care) have responsibility for a safe discharge and for identifying continuing health and social care needs. They will generate a referral to the relevant social services department or other agencies. Many hospitals also have specialist nurses (eg. discharge liaison nurse or 'care management facilitator') who will assist with particularly complex cases.

Trigger questions for housing staff

- Do you know the hospitals in your area and which NHS trusts run them?

- Are you confident that housing issues are highlighted in hospital discharge policies?

- Have you made it your business to inform the hospitals about your agency or department's housing policies, priority and allocation systems, etc?

- Do you have an officer whose task it is to liaise on hospital discharge?

- Do appropriate housing staff liaise regularly with local hospitals?

- Do you have a contact name and number for the hospital discharge liaison nurse or equivalent in the hospitals you deal with?

- Have you sent these hospitals details of the services of your agency/department with contact names and numbers?

- Do you have contact names and numbers for social services workers responsible for discharge in the hospitals you deal with?

General issues for operational staff from the agencies involved in hospital discharge

Issue

Housing needs
The housing needs of patients are rarely included in the requirements of hospital discharge policies. This dimension is essential for an effective care plan and discharge procedure and needs to be attended to as soon as possible after admission to hospital.

Involvement of housing agency staff
Involvement of housing departments and agencies in the discharge planning process is relatively rare.

Lack of knowledge and understanding
Awareness among hospital staff and social services staff of the housing status and needs of patients being considered for admission and discharge is viewed by many housing workers as insufficient.

There can be a lack of knowledge among hospital social services and health staff about housing, housing options and priorities and, between health, social services and housing agencies, a lack of shared understanding of each other's cultures.

What needs to be done and by whom

Hospital management and social services staff
A multi-disciplinary care assessment should include housing need. Hospital discharge policies must be reviewed and this omission remedied in consultation with representatives of housing agencies. The Health Authority can be requested to act on this if necessary.

Hospital management and social services staff
A housing representative or a person responsible for liaison between housing and hospital and social services staff should be involved in discharge planning discussions which have a housing dimension.

Hospital and social services staff and housing department staff
Regular joint seminars and workshops could focus on the housing dimensions of hospital admission and discharge and on how discharge looks from both the hospital and the community perspective. This should be incorporated in routine training.

Responsibility for positive outreach and networking from one setting to another should be placed with named individuals and should be preserved where possible in the context of staff turnover.

Equally, it is difficult for housing agency staff to understand the urgency of delayed discharge and to appreciate the risks involved for frail or elderly persons of prolonged stays in hospitals.

Practical pressures and realities
Hospital staff are under great pressure to prevent prolonged hospital stays and to respond to rising numbers of emergency admissions, waiting list targets, etc. It is difficult for hospital staff to understand the practical realities of arranging care, support and housing at short notice in the community and the pressures on other agencies.

Building up a body of knowledge
Extremely complex discharge cases with a housing dimension are a minority of the discharges from the average acute hospital. Hospital-based staff do not therefore easily build up a body of routine knowledge and contacts re housing.

Information
Hospital-based staff frequently have to liaise with a number of local authorities and large catchment areas. It is difficult for them to know where to find information about housing.

Homelessness
Hospital-based staff often have a poor understanding of definitions of 'homelessness' and thus sometimes fail to activate the speediest route to housing on discharge. Patients themselves are not always able to supply full information if unprompted by staff.

Housing agency staff
Managers could include training about hospital discharge at induction and updates.

Social services and housing
An intermediary could be jointly appointed whose job it is to facilitate understanding and collaboration between the parties involved.
This intermediary should draw in housing agency staff to participate in admission and discharge planning procedures involving housing.

Housing departments
Local authorities could set up one central point of information in local housing departments via which enquiries may be routed. This should also cover information about housing agencies with available accommodation.

Housing departments could provide their local hospitals with a simple directory of local housing services and responsibilities. This should contain a clear statement of housing priorities and details of the distribution of housing functions (including the meaning of technical terms and departmental labels). The directory should have named contacts and phone numbers.

Social services and housing
Need to address this issue and train those concerned with admission and discharge. A checklist of criteria on homelessness for use at ward level should be mutually agreed (see example of good practice).

Every local authority is required to have a designated person to make assessments with regard to homelessness. In small authorities, these may not be in housing departments but in environmental health or another department. Dedicated homeless persons teams may be attached to housing departments or to healthcare trusts.

Services in sheltered housing

Assumptions are sometimes made by hospital staff that personal care and support services for individuals can be expected from the wardens of sheltered housing where they are resident.

Loss of tenancy in sheltered housing

Patients are sometimes persuaded to give up the tenancy of their sheltered accommodation precipitatively in the view of hospital staff.

Occupational therapy assessments

Occupational therapy assessments are one element in the total needs assessment of an individual. The occupational therapist's appraisal of the individual's functional capacity in the home situation needs also to be set in the total environment so that referrals can be made where more extensive repairs are needed.

Hospital/community occupational therapists

The fact that occupational therapists are employed separately by hospitals and by community social services can be an impediment to a smooth process of hospital discharge and suitable housing adaptations and options. The shortage of community occupational therapists in many areas also leads to long waiting lists and long delays in housing adaptations, and yet occupational therapy assessments are often pivotal to hospital discharge planning.

Retention of the house while in hospital

The consequences of an unplanned admission for a person who lives alone may be serious. If no one is paying the rent or if an insecure house is vandalised or squatters move in, this may lead to the loss of a home. The neglect or abandonment of pets may cause additional stress to the patient.

Hospital and social services staff

The inability (and lack of training) of wardens to provide such services needs to form part of regular input to training of hospital-based staff.

Registered social landlords

Some registered social landlords send a printed card in to the hospital with the resident, making clear the limitations of their facilities and wardens in relation to medical and personal care and support needs. For an example of this, see below.

Registered social landlords

Decisions about tenancy should be a part of the assessment process. Registered social landlords should give notice in written form to tenants.

Housing's educational role

There is a need for good communications and exchange between occupational therapists, the local authority section dealing with grants for home repair and improvement, and where they exist, Home Improvement Agencies (See **Module Four**.)

Health and social services

In some areas, hospital and community occupational therapists have been joined to form one service and to improve continuity between hospital and home.

Ward staff and hospital social services

Ward staff need to make early enquiries about a lone individual's home circumstances and alert social services for appropriate action. Community mental health teams or housing support workers may also be able to help with these urgent problems.

Returning home
The risk that a patient will be discharged to a cold and empty house needs to be avoided.

Ward staff and hospital social services
Ward staff need to make early enquiries about a lone individual's home circumstances and alert social services for appropriate action by the homecare service to turn on heating and make other preparations.

Example of good practice

Information on hospital admission

....

is a resident of _____ housing association warden-assisted accommodation. The warden is available (not necessarily on site) on a 24-hour basis to ensure the safety and security of residents.

Should personal care and support services be required on discharge from hospital, normal community care services should be arranged.

Suggestions for good practice

Local contact sheet for housing agency staff

The key individuals involved in hospital discharge are:

- the consultant;

- the named nurse on the patient's ward in the hospital;

- the clinical nurse specialist (eg, discharge liaison nurse or care management facilitator);

- the relevant social worker (eg, hospital or community social worker);

- other members of the multi-disciplinary team (eg, the hospital occupational therapist, physiotherapist, etc);

- hospital transport;

- the patient's GP;

- the district or community nurse or health visitor (contact local health centre or clinic);

- locality social services (care manager, social worker, occupational therapist, home care organiser, Meals on Wheels organiser).

Housing agency staff may like to adapt the following to their requirements:

Local hospitals	Key contacts	Tel:
Community and primary healthcare		
Social services	Key contacts	Tel:

Trigger questions on pre-admission or admission for health and social services staff (ward level and Accident and Emergency)

[For the admitting nurse, nurse responsible for care and social worker]

1   What information does the patient need?

2   Does the patient just admitted

   • live alone?
   • require arrangements to be made for paying rent?
   • require arrangements to be made for securing her property?
   • require arrangements to be made for safeguarding/feeding a pet?
   • require arrangements for turning the heating on prior to discharge?

3   Do housing/social services support workers need to be contacted to deal with any of these problems?

4   Does the patient want to return to their previous home or to an alternative kind of accommodation? Is there any risk to the patient returning to previous accommodation?

5   Is the patient to be discharged likely to need

   • aids and equipment?
   • minor adaptations?
   • major adaptations?
   • housing renovation?
   • alternative housing?

6   What is the housing tenure of the patient to be discharged?

   • owner-occupier?
   • private tenant?
   • housing association tenant?
   • council tenant?
   • homeless?

7   Has the patient enough money for discharge?

8   Does the patient need to be referred to community health services or to social services?

9   Does the patient need to clarify their benefit entitlement with the Benefits Agency?

10 Do representatives of the housing department/housing association need to be contacted?

11 Does the designated homeless persons officer (housing department)/ homeless persons team (Health Authority/NHS trust/housing department/voluntary agency) need to be contacted? (See discharge planning map opposite.)

From hospital to home
Housing action required in discharge planning
Question: is this chart an accurate representation of typical pathways in your area?
Suggestion: if not, it might serve as a model for you to map them?

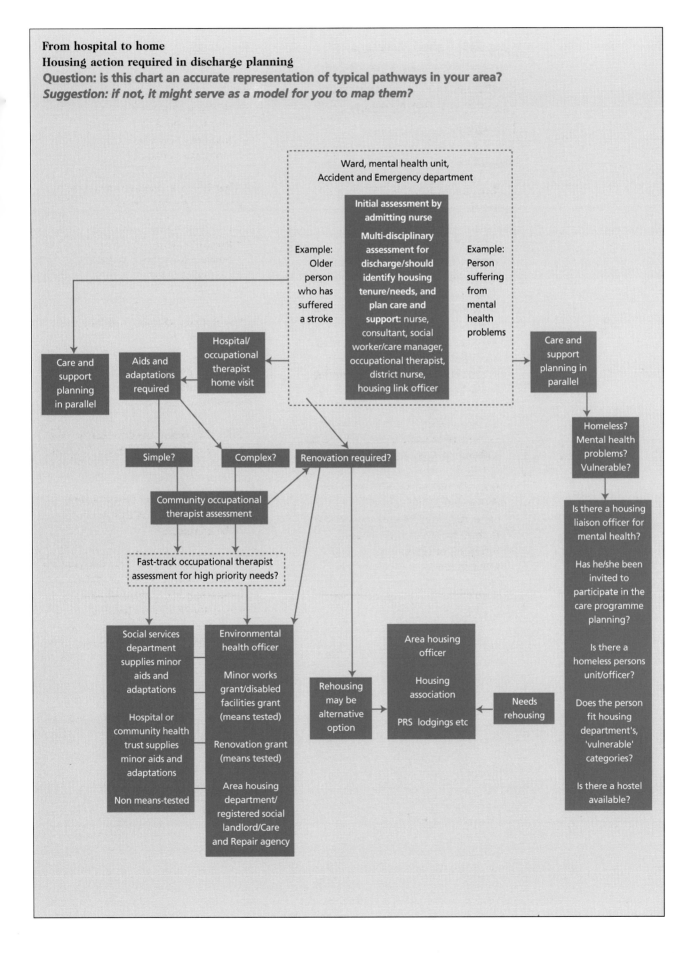

Care and Repair/housing renovation for private sector tenants and owner-occupiers

Anchor Hospital Discharge Project, London Borough of Hackney

What is Anchor Hospital Discharge?

Anchor Hospital Discharge is run by the Anchor Trust and funded by the local Health Authority.

The service is targeted at older and disabled people living in the private sector who have been admitted to either the Homerton or Hackney hospitals and who normally live in the London Borough of Hackney. The project aims to give advice, practical help and support to older and disabled people who are having difficulties being discharged from hospital due to their housing conditions.

Specialist welfare rights advice and help with grant applications is provided by the project staff. Assistance can be given with finding temporary accommodation whilst work is carried out on a client's home.

After referral, the Project staff will endeavour to keep all services informed of progress.

Professional and technical advice and assistance in rectifying property defects and organising adaptations to the client's home will be provided. Assistance will also be provided in securing the necessary funding for the work.

Making a referral

As soon as a client in hospital is seen to have a problem with their home conditions the professional involved, either social worker, nurse, doctor or occupational therapist should ring the project to make a referral. Referral forms are available. *An early referral will reduce delays.*

After referral a caseworker will visit the client in hospital and make an initial assessment to discover their needs and wishes. The caseworker is there to act as the client's support worker during the whole process of planning and executing any building works. Continuous support will be given until the client is settled back into their home.

The caseworker will discuss the client's needs with the technical officer and will then do a home visit either with the client or with an appropriate professional involved or a relative.

The technical officer will advise on the schedule of works to be undertaken. The caseworker will inform the client, relatives and professionals involved, what can be undertaken in the home, what funding could be available, and the possible timescale. In every case there may not be an ideal solution and the caseworker will advise on temporary and long term solutions to housing problems.

The technical officer will provide drawings and specifications for any work needed and will obtain estimates from reliable builders from our approved list of building and specialist contractors.

The caseworker will process any grant applications for the works and will keep in close contact with the environmental health department as to the progress of any applications. The caseworker will also give advice about other sources of finance where a grant is not available.

Once funding has been agreed the technical officer will oversee and inspect the work at all stages until satisfactory completion. Where building work is carried out, a fee for technical services provided will be levied. If a client is eligible for a grant the fee is included in the grant. No fee is charged for caseworker support services.

Contact: Project Manager, Anchor Hospital Discharge, 133 Stoke Newington High Street, London N16 0PH, Tel: 0171 241 0632

Ward level assessment and care planning for discharge of homeless people

[A section taken from Patient Care Documentation, University College London Hospitals]

Accommodation		*Please check with patient/carer or relevant housing personnel first as to whether:*
(Prior to admission)		1. Patient can return to this accommodation on discharge
Owner-occupied	☐	2. Accommodation is suitable for patient to return to eg, heating, facilities, access or any risk to patient
Rented	☐	
Residential/nursing home	☐	If answer **No/Unsure** to either question above, **refer to Discharge linkworker** (see below)
Sheltered/supported housing	☐	
Living with friends/relatives	☐	
No fixed abode/squat	☐	**Refer to Discharge linkworker**
Hostel	☐	
Bed & Breakfast	☐	Tel: Bleep:
Temporary accommodation	☐	

Homelessness assessment sheet for use at ward level

[A section taken from Patient Care Documentation, University College London Hospitals]

Name _____	GP name _____
Address _____	Address _____
_____	_____
_____	_____
_____	_____
_____	
Religion _____	Admission date _____
DOB _____	
	Planned discharge date _____
Ward _____	
Consultant _____	
Specialty _____	
Originator _____	

Ward: Assessment Sheet: HOMELESS PERSONS DISCHARGE

REFER TO GUIDELINES [ ] Anticipated discharge date [_____]
Named nurse: [_____]
Local authority patient pre-admission: [_____]

Do you think priority housing is needed [ ] If yes, referred to:
[_____]
If other borough, please state: _____

_____

Name of social worker/care manager: [_____]
Name of homeless persons unit officer [_____]
Date of referral: [_____]

Discharge destination: [_____]
If other, please state: [_____]
[_____]   Is patient registered with GP: [ ]
If no, registration/care details given: [ ]

Is patient receiving benefit: [ ]   If no, referred to: [_____]
If yes, referred for further advice: [_____]
[_____] Is medical certificate required: [ ]
Has patient enough money for discharge? [ ] If no, referred to: [_____]
[_____]

'NOTES' advice sheet in medical notes? [ ] Are all care plan details completed? [ ]
Actual discharge date [_____]
Name/status of discharging nurse: [_____]

Housing issues for health and social services staff dealing with hospital discharge of people with mental health problems

Social services are obliged under Section 47 of the 1990 Health and Community Care Act to assess the needs of individuals for community care services and, where necessary, to do this in collaboration with housing authorities and others.

More frequently than is the case for other patients, discharge of people with mental health problems (which could be from a psychiatric ward, from a general ward or from an accident and emergency department) will involve housing problems and homelessness, sometimes exacerbated by drug or alcohol misuse. A full understanding of the category of 'homelessness' is often lacking in the discharge process.

Frequently, representatives of housing agencies become involved in joint needs assessment only in cases of severe housing need such as *street homelessness*. It is reported by housing officers that their input tends to be after the assessment and relates to the preparation or allocation of property. "This suggests that lead authority assessors have limited perceptions of what constitutes housing need and thus take little account of housing need." (Cardiff Housing Department)

The definition of homelessness

Homelessness is not just street homelessness. People are homeless if they live in hostels, bed and breakfast accommodation, use night shelters, are squatting, or are temporarily living with friends or relatives.

Under the homeless persons legislation, applicants must fall into one of the 'priority' groups in order to be considered for rehousing under the provisions of the Act. Priority need includes being the victim of fire, flood or other disaster or being vulnerable due to old age, mental illness, learning disability, physical impairment or major health problem.

Local housing authorities have specific accommodation responsibilities to those homeless people who are homeless, in priority need and have no suitable accommodation available to them. Priority can come from being vulnerable because of mental illness. Allocation of a local authority secure tenancy or nomination for a registered social landlord assured tenancy must be via obtaining sufficient priority on the housing register.

Key points

It is vital

- that housing agencies should be brought into the assessment and care management process;

- that hospital patients with accommodation needs should be referred to housing departments *at admission stage*, whether or not community care needs are indicated;

- that joint training should be implemented for all staff involved in the assessment and discharge planning process;

- to the success of maintaining tenancies that housing staff are notified of the care packages to be provided and are supplied with a named contact;

- to remember that the provision of inadequate support will undermine the confidence of housing providers in the assessment and discharge process.

Many people discharged from psychiatric and mental handicap hospitals and local authority hostels into the community may be regarded as vulnerable. Health Authorities have an express duty under advice contained in DH circulars (90)23 and LASSL(90)11 to implement a specifically tailored care programme for all patients considered for discharge from psychiatric hospitals and all new patients accepted by the specialist psychiatric services. (London Housing Unit, 1996)

Basic principles of the Care Programme Approach

Department of Health Circular 'The Care Programme Approach for people with a mental illness referred to specialist psychiatric services' (HC(90)23/ LASSL(90)11) required Health Authorities to implement the Care Programme Approach (CPA) for all patients accepted for specialist psychiatric services, particularly those with severe and continuing mental illness. The core elements of the CPA are:

• systematic assessment of health and social care needs;

• an agreed programme of care drawn up to address these needs;

• nominated key workers;

• regular reviews.

Suitable housing will be required to complement some care programmes. Where this is the case, early involvement of the housing authority is crucial so that suitable arrangements can be incorporated into the care programme. Health Authorities should ensure that arrangements for implementing the CPA include discussions with social services and housing about housing and support services.

Housing questions for health and social services staff dealing with hospital discharge

1   How are the housing needs of the patient addressed in the care plan?

2   Has the local authority housing department been invited and given sufficient notice to participate in the housing needs assessment of those with mental health problems?

3   Does the local authority housing department have a specially designated mental health liaison officer or other specific arrangements for assisting in the housing needs assessment of those with mental health problems (eg, multi-disciplinary mental health panel)?

4   Do the relevant health and social services staff have the necessary information on housing availability and housing agencies?

Hospital discharge issues for housing agency staff

Housing departments and homeless persons units are sometimes faced with "situations where homeless people with mental health problems have been discharged with little or no advance warning at reception areas and with nowhere to stay. This has caused some tension between local authority Housing Departments and Health Authorities, although it has been successfully addressed in some localities". (London Housing Unit, 1996)

Common problems include:

• housing authorities tend to reject for rehousing short-term psychiatric patients discharged from hospital because the health (trust) no longer classifies them as *vulnerable*;

• housing authorities and agencies have been reluctant to take on vulnerable people discharged from short stay institutions when they present themselves without a package of care from the health (trust), since they are perceived as potential housing management problems.

Homelessness code of guidance for local authorities

Wherever possible housing authorities should identify a nominated homelessness liaison officer to liaise between the department dealing with housing and Health Authorities or departments on, for example, the rehousing of patients on discharge from NHS general, psychiatric and mental handicap hospitals and hostels. Authorities will, however, need to be aware that these arrangements sometimes fall down and should be sensitive to direct approaches from discharged patients who are homeless. (London Housing Unit, 1996)

A checklist of questions for housing workers follows. Reference should also be made to the section of **Module Two** relating to 'mapping healthcare' and p 110 of this module on 'trigger questions on admission for health and social services staff'.

Mental health checklist for housing workers

1 Do you know how to contact your local:

• Mental health team?
• Social services departments?
• Neighbourhood beat officer?
• Mental health advocacy centre?
• Users/self-help group?
• Mental health charity centres?
• Citizens Advice Bureau?

2 Do you know what to do if:

• You suspect someone has a mental health problem?
• Someone you suspect has mental health problems is not paying their rent or causing other housing administration difficulties?
• Neighbours complain about the behaviour of a person with mental health problems?
• There is a violent incident involving someone in mental distress in your neighbourhood office or on the estate?

3 Have you received interview and communication skills training?

4 Do you have access to mental health literature and someone to discuss mental health problems with?

5 Do you have a referrals and assessment procedure with your local mental health teams?

6 Do you know how to set up a service delivery package with other community services?

Source: Thompson et al (1995)

Example of good practice

Inter-agency working on discharges from Whitchurch Hospital, Cardiff

Background

In partnership with health and social services, an innovative discharge procedure has been introduced in Cardiff by the housing department in order to process homelessness applications from people leaving Whitchurch Hospital, a hospital which provides for people with mental health problems. The procedure acknowledges the need for the early involvement of the housing department by requesting information about people who may be in housing need at the point of admission to hospital. The procedure has been in operation since January 1995 and the housing department allocated access to 20 units of accommodation for a period of one year; it is the access to the accommodation which is designated rather than the bricks and mortar.

Accommodation

For those people who are not considered vulnerable, the housing department has no duty to rehouse them. However, in these cases, advice and assistance can be provided to ensure that planned accommodation is available on discharge.

This service is also provided to people who do not wish to present as homeless or who wish to access private sector accommodation.

Support

Prior to allocating accommodation to those people considered as vulnerable, an inter-agency meeting is held to ensure that an adequate support package is in place and that particular housing need is addressed. Details of the key worker responsible for coordinating the support are given to the estate manager responsible for the management of the tenancy, so that ongoing liaison can take place.

Procedure overview

Admission

A pro forma is used by hospital ward managers to collect information on a fortnightly basis on all admissions to hospital where accommodation is an issue. This pro forma, which includes details of the named nurse and the expected discharge date, is forwarded to a named housing officer.

Assessment

An assessment of housing and support needs is carried out within a timescale suggested by the likely discharge date. This housing assessment is conducted by the hospital from which the individual was discharged is contacted for clarification and discharge. Once this is received appropriate section is taken; such action varies from case to case.

Monitoring

In order to assess the success of the procedure a form was distributed to housing officers, housing agencies, hostels and following action by the housing agency concerned, the completed notification form is forwarded to the Health Authority purchasing team responsible for mental assessment of support needs is made by a named social worker drawn from the community mental health team.

For further details of this initative, contact the community care development officer at Cardiff Coutny Council, Telephone: 01222 822221

(*Welsh Housing Quarterly*, Issue 22, 1996)

Guide to further reading

Barnes, M. and Cormie, J. (1995) 'Hospital discharge: on the panel', *Health Service Journal*, 2 March.

Clark, H., Dyer, S. and Hartman, L. (1996) *Going home: older people leaving hospital*, Bristol: The Policy Press. [A study of the experiences of older people being discharged from hospital, especially those needing housing adaptations and/or special equipment.]

Goss, S. and Kent, C. (1995) *Health and housing: working together? A review of inter-agency working*, Bristol: The Policy Press. [Barriers are identified, good practice examples given and factor likely to promote joint working are highlighted.]

Health Advisory Service (1995) *A place in mind: commissioning and providing mental health services for people who are homeless*, London: HMSO. [Covers operational as well as strategic issues.]

Henwood, M. (1994) *Hospital discharge workbook: a manual on hospital discharge practice*, London: Department of Health. [Designed to promote good discharge both from the point of view of patients and professionals.]

Henwood, M. (1994), 'Going by the book', *Health Service Journal*, 31 March.

Hudson, B. (1996) 'Health, housing, hiatus', *Health Service Journal*, 20 June.

London Housing Unit (1996) *Being there: tenants with mental health support needs: an analysis of working practices in London*. LHU, Bedford House, 125-133 Camden High St. London NW1 7JR.

Thompson, K. et al (1995) *Mental health care: a guide for housing workers*, London: Mental Health Foundation. [This guide is targeted at the needs of housing workers and includes coverage of the legislation; how mental health services are organised, the importance of joint working and common questions.]